Praise for
calm **mama** happy **baby**

"At last, a book *for* moms (and dads) *about* the moms (and dads) of babies! *Calm Mama, Happy Baby* presents an individualized road map for navigating the often stressful and sometimes shaky first years of parenthood. Derek O'Neill and Jennifer Waldburger clearly understand the symbiotic relationship between parent and child and the emotional rollercoaster ride that is parenting. Their hands-on tool kit, filled with specific tips for coping with the early parenting journey, is a must for every parent's library."

—**Betsy Brown Braun, MA**
Child development and behavior specialist
Author of *Just Tell Me What to Say* and *You're Not the Boss of Me*

"As a mom, I have absolutely found a connection between my stress or calm and my daughter's mood and behavior. *Calm Mama, Happy Baby* gives moms fun and practical tools for choosing calm over stress no matter what is happening with their child. These techniques have been a lifesaver for me."

—**Tiffani Thiessen, actress**

"When we adopted our daughter, I immediately sought information on how to nurture a healthy attachment. *Calm Mama, Happy Baby is* a must-read for helping parents build a foundation of trust, security, and connection to help their baby thrive."

—**Nia Vardalos, actress and writer,** "My Big Fat Greek Wedding"
Author of *New York Times* bestseller *Instant Mom*

"New parents are inundated with advice on 'the right way' to raise a child. As a pediatrician and father, I have seen firsthand how information overload, even if well intentioned, can lead to stress and anxiety for a new parent. *Calm Mama, Happy Baby* helps parents deal with stress and create a positive environment for themselves and their child. Happy parents definitely make happier babies."

—**Scott Cohen, MD, FAAP**
Author of *Eat, Sleep, Poop: A Common Sense Guide to Your Baby's First Year*
Co-founder, Beverly Hills Pediatrics

"A fascinating look at how we are neurologically 'programmed' to think, feel, and act like our parents. This book shows moms how to avoid passing along habits of stress and negativity, setting their children up for good health, optimal learning, and better sleep."

—**Anjalee Warrier Galion, MD**
Assistant Program Director, Child Neurology Training Program
Children's Hospital of Orange County

"Kids raised in calm households tend to fare better academically, emotionally, socially, and physically. *Calm Mama, Happy Baby* helps parents live more peaceful—and therefore healthier—lives, and the benefits to their child are immeasurable."

—**Sonya Sethi Gohill, MD, FAAP**
Founder, Brentwood Pediatrics
Attending pediatrician, Cedars-Sinai Medical Center and St. John's Health Center

"After countless classes and books on sleep, we knew it was time to call in the big guns, so we called Jen. Who knew that it was worry and anxiety about our two-year-old not sleeping that was actually contributing to her wakefulness? After using the principles in *Calm Mama, Happy Baby*, we went from bumpy nights to peaceful ones. We are true believers now!"

—**Erin Lokitz and Tony Kanal, musician**

"Finally! A book that addresses what I've always observed: calm and happy parents tend to have calmer and happier children, and stressed-out parents tend to have more stressed-out children. *Calm Mama, Happy Baby* offers simple tools for managing the stress and worry that come with being a parent. I look forward to recommending this book to my families to help ensure that their child has the best possible start in life."

—**Bess Raker, MD**
Co-founder, Beverly Hills Pediatrics
Attending pediatrician, Cedars-Sinai Medical Center

"As a psychiatrist specializing in postpartum depression, I am so grateful to have a resource that offers step-by-step guidelines for how to manage the ups and downs of being a new parent. By helping moms tap into their natural instincts with confidence, and respond mindfully to their newborns, this book makes the transition to parenthood a much more peaceful experience."

—**Stephanie Zisook, MD**
Reproductive psychiatrist, UCLA Clinical Faculty

"Attachment Parenting begins with listening to your baby, and this book helps parents with that in every way. It's pretty easy to miss your baby's cues if you're a new parent awakened every hour or two. *Calm Mama, Happy Baby* is great reading and helps us understand our babies' needs and form the close, loving bond we all want."

—**Jay Gordon, MD**
Author of *Good Nights: The Happy Parents' Guide to the Family Bed*

"Evolving into motherhood has been a journey for me, and this guidance has been so instrumental. When I get stressed, I just keep thinking, 'calm mama happy baby.'"

—**Kristen, mom of Brody, 2 months**

"When I take a deep breath and the baby settles, it's a 'wow.'"

—**Lauren, mom of Amelie, 4 months**

"As a type-A mom who puts a lot of pressure on herself to be the best mom possible, I sometimes forget to breathe, let my shoulders down, and relax, but this book is a good reminder that being calm helps not only mom but baby, too. As a new mom, being calm is all you can do when you realize you don't have control."

—**Robin, mom of Jackson, 9 months**

"I am incredibly hard on myself and have such all-or-nothing thoughts about my success or failure as a mother. This book gave me permission to trust my own heart and instincts."

—**Alyssa, mom of Talia, 6 months**

"Doing the deep breathing and staying calm while putting my baby to bed has had a huge impact on his ability to settle. I am feeling much more positive about bedtime in our house!"

—**Alexis, mom of Desmond, 5 months**

"I really love the baby's reaction when I take deep breaths—it stops him in his tracks. So does talking to him in a calm voice. My biggest takeaway from this book is to be aware that when Kyle's little upsets do arise, I can take a look at myself first and make any adjustments."

—Lisa, mom of Kyle, 12 months

"As I read this book, I felt like you were sitting with me on my couch and addressing everything I am going through as a new mom with laser precision. Thank you!"

—Jenna, mom of Sidney, 4 months

calm **mama**
happy **baby**

The Simple, Intuitive Way
to Tame Tears, Improve Sleep,
and Help Your Family Thrive

Derek O'Neill, CHP, and
Jennifer Waldburger, MSW
Coauthor of The Sleepeasy Solution

Health Communications, Inc.
Deerfield Beach, Florida

www.hcibooks.com

**The Library of Congress Cataloging-in-Publication Data
is available through the Library of Congress**

© 2013 Derek O'Neill and Jennifer Waldburger

ISBN-13: 978-0-7573-1766-8 (paperback)
ISBN-10: 0-7573-1766-9 (paperback)
ISBN-13: 978-0-7573-1767-5 (ePub)
ISBN-10: 0-7573-1767-7 (ePub)

Publisher: Health Communications, Inc.
      3201 S.W. 15th Street
      Deerfield Beach, FL 33442-8190

Cover photo ©Ariana Falerni, www.arianafalerni.com
Cover design by Larissa Hise Henoch
Interior design and formatting by Lawna Patterson Oldfield

This book is dedicated to
the memory of Linda O'Neill,
whose calm, loving presence is a
living legacy that continues to bring
peace and joy to all whose
lives she touched.

Contents

Foreword

For many years, I had the privilege and joy of taking care of thousands of babies and kids—and parents, too—in my pediatric practice. A new baby brings incredible joy to a family, but being a parent is stressful, too. These days, with many parents working outside of the home, the influx of too much information on the Internet, and conflicting advice hitting new parents from all directions, staying calm is a difficult challenge, even under the best of circumstances.

My favorite expression in practice was that "Great Danes give birth to Great Danes, and Chihuahuas to Chihuahuas." Not only do babies typically look like their parents, but they also acquire the persona and personality traits of the people who surround them from the time they take their first breath. In my observation, it was always apparent early on that those parents (and especially moms) who were calm, empowered, and natural problem-solvers *before* the baby was born usually continued to be so after delivery, too. After meeting their extended families and the baby's grandparents, I could often see that the trend of calm energy flowed through the generations, and these babies were raised in a peaceful environment with a minimum of hardship. Even when there were challenges, these families seemed remarkably resilient, able to flex and adapt to what came their way. Children of these calmer parents often seemed to follow suit.

What was also very apparent was that parents who were either overtly nervous or anxious, or who acted calm and organized but were a bundle of nerves inside at the first sign of trouble, had a very different experience than calmer moms and dads. These more frustrated parents often had a harder time accessing problem-solving skills when their baby was crying, as their personal stress prevented them from objectively assessing what their baby needed. Once again, the children followed suit; these little ones fussed more and often grew into kids who had a hard time rolling with the ups and downs of life unless I intervened with supportive options. I typically referred these families to the parent groups conducted by Jennifer and Derek—my trusted go-to experts to help parents achieve a better balance for themselves and, as a result, for their babies.

Whether you're calmer or more stressed by nature, though, as a parent you want what's best for your baby, and you're doing the best that you can. Every mom has moments when the you-know-what hits the fan unexpectedly, and every mom can benefit from learning better ways to manage stress. *Calm Mama, Happy Baby* will show you how, with simple, step-by-step supports that are easy to use and lean on. What Jen and Derek have done is to give moms—and all parents, as well as caregivers—a powerful set of tools to recognize when personal stress gets in the way of loving connection, healthy attachment, and effective intervention with their babies. All can be achieved from the comfort of your couch!

Using the acronym "CALM," in this book you will learn how to:

*C*ancel *negative thoughts* and clear away distracting mind chatter;

*A*llow *your feelings* and manage your emotions so that your perspective on your baby's needs is accurate and realistic;

*L*ink *up and listen* by tuning in to the subtle aspects of your baby's communication, so you can problem solve and attend to her more effectively; and

*M*irror and empathize appropriately with your baby so she feels safe and loved no matter what she's experiencing.

The CALM method and other support tools offered in this book allow parents to accurately assess even the most challenging situations with their baby in just a few moments. Feeling more empowered to trust their own intuition, moms can then respond to their child with confidence and clarity rather than reacting with anxiety and distress.

I would certainly recommend that parents read this book *before* your baby is born so you can develop trust in yourself and build skills early to feel more prepared for the wonderful but daunting task of becoming a parent. And if you've already welcomed a baby and would like to begin feeling more calm and centered right now, shoot straight to Chapter 3 and dive in.

Using the principles and supports in this book will help you give your baby a healthy, happy start in life. My thanks to Jen and Derek for providing a much-needed resource for parents who truly want to offer the best they can to their child.

JJ Levenstein, MD, FAAP
Retired pediatrician, founder of Boulevard Pediatrics
President and cofounder of MD MOMS
Pediatric instructor at MomAssembly.com

Preface

You've been awake since 3:27 AM, when the baby roused you out of what we could call sleep but more closely resembles an altered state of consciousness. Jolted into instantaneous full alert, you are like a firefighter ready for action: Shaking off your fatigue, you arrive on the scene, prepared to do whatever it takes to put out the fire. You pick up the crying baby, who feels hot and damp, and offer shushes and soft words of reassurance so as not to wake your sleeping husband.* (Just how *can* he sleep through this wailing, anyway?) Making your way quickly to the glider, you position the baby and offer the breast. You're still new at this, but even in your exhausted state, somehow you seem to know exactly how to respond. Within seconds, your crying baby is the picture of calm, happily guzzling away. Your own breathing starts to regulate, though your heart is still beating with the *thump-thump* of a mother's worry about her child's well-being. Gazing at her now, satisfied by her sounds of sucking and her closed, sleepy eyes, you can finally relax; you have responded to your baby, and she calmed—*this time.***

---

* Throughout this book, we refer to a mom's partner as male as a matter of grammatical convenience only.

** For convenience, the pronoun *she* is used throughout this book to refer to a baby.

It doesn't always go exactly like that, though. Sometimes your baby cries—and cries, and cries, and cries, even after a feeding and a diaper change, a burp, and being rocked, bounced, swung, and swaddled. Sometimes you can't fix it; no matter what you try, pulling out every trick in your brand-new bag, you can't seem to help her settle. And then you panic. You feel like a failure, and you beat yourself up. *What's wrong with me?*, you think. *Why can't I calm my baby? What am I missing, and why don't I know what to do?* The more the baby cries, the more anxious you feel, and the more anxious you feel, the more she cries. Finally, almost an hour later, she might pass out from sheer exhaustion, falling into an agitated sleep that lasts as little as twenty minutes before she's up again, still unsettled and needing more help. At that point, you feel like crying yourself.

As a mom, when you respond to your child and she calms, you believe in yourself. You believe in nature and your instincts, and you feel the forces of the universe flowing through you and supporting every move you make. You are in sync with a grand plan that involves both you and your baby, and all is well. But when you respond to your child and she doesn't calm, you berate yourself. You believe you have let her down, that you have missed the mark. You feel the weight of the universe on your shoulders, and you want to give up—or throw up—in response to all the pressure to be a "good mother," whatever that means. You want to give the baby to another mother who could do a better job, who could do the right thing, because you can't, and you don't even know what that right thing is. You feel sharp pangs of anxiety and are frustrated beyond measure, but you share these feelings with a very select few, if anyone, because you believe you're the only mom who has them. Too many moms seem to dance between believing that they're failing miserably and believing that *maybe,* just maybe, they're doing well enough.

The most important ingredient in a mother's intention as she attends to her child, her innate sense of what's best—what we commonly think of as "mother's instinct"—really boils down to one thing: trust. Not trust in the Internet, the parenting books, the Mommy and Me leaders, the pediatricians, or even extended family and other mom friends, but trust in *herself*. A mom who trusts herself knows that even when she takes in information from outside sources, she can sense, intuitively, whether that information is right for her baby. The question is, how does she find that trust given that she's navigating unfamiliar waters as a new mom? In our work with mothers over the years—whether in therapy sessions, new-mom groups, or seminars—we've found that the answer to that question rests in a choice: to buy into the idea that you're getting it wrong as a mom, which causes lots of stress and disconnects you from your mama instincts, or to center yourself in the belief that doing your best is not only good enough but an act of tremendous love and service to your baby. When you believe in yourself as a mom, you not only enjoy a healthier attachment to your baby and a stronger sense of intuition about what she needs but also a more positive, peaceful parenting experience.

Staying grounded in the midst of diaper blowouts, bedtime battles, and the vortex that is daily family life isn't easy. Derek, a dad who admittedly wasn't always calm while raising his own kids, knows this firsthand, and Jennifer, a "mom to many" through her work, is no stranger to stress and anxiety herself. So we get it, though

> When you believe in yourself as a mom, you not only enjoy a healthier attachment to your baby and a stronger sense of intuition about what she needs but also a more positive, peaceful parenting experience.

please know that we're entering the picture here not as experts about you or your child, because that's your domain. Instead, we are two people who have been listening to your stories about motherhood for more than four decades, from both personal and professional vantage points, and we'd like to offer some support and insights that may be useful or helpful.

Throughout this book, our aim is to help you deepen your trust and faith in your abilities as a mom. We'll also help you explore what zaps your energy the most, and we'll show you how to dissolve the blocks that prevent you from accessing your intuition as a mom. We'll offer some simple processes—designed for busy moms who don't have lots of time—that will help you to handle stress and negativity when they come and to enjoy a deeper, more peaceful connection with yourself, your baby, and others. But please don't just take the ideas we offer in this book at face value. Test-drive them, try them on, and stretch and bend them, adapting as you see fit; discover for yourself what resonates and what doesn't. We're not the experts on what works best for you, you are.

Whether you feel stressed and overwhelmed on a daily basis or whether you're a fairly calm mama who'd just like to feel that way even more than you already do, we look forward to helping you enjoy life more, not only as a mom but as a multifaceted person with her own interests, needs, and dreams. Here's to honoring and celebrating all that you are.

CHAPTER 1

Little **Bright** Lights

A s you well know, you have a very aware little being living under your roof. From an early age—perhaps even since birth—your child has appeared incredibly alert, missing nothing as she takes in information from her environment. Her sharp senses cause her to be amazingly responsive to the sights and sounds around her; to her, there is never a dull moment. She may also not care much about sleeping or eating, despite your concerns on either front, as she's got better things to do. Your child is so awake, in fact, that people comment on this often, along with her wide-open eyes and extremely focused gaze.

Just who *is* this extraordinary little person who has come into your life? Of course, all parents like to believe that their child is unusually intelligent—this has always been so—but the children coming into the world these days really do seem remarkably bright. They don't just seem intelligent, they seem far *more* intelligent than we are, and highly advanced. Some are rolling, crawling, and walking much earlier than they typically would at their age; others are on a fast track cognitively, seeming to understand not only every word you say but even what you *don't* say. The babies being born these days also seem incredibly resilient and happy; despite sometimes having strong reactions to life's bumpy road while they adjust to being here in the first few months of life, as they grow they tend to recover from their ups and downs very quickly. If it weren't for the disguise of their very small bodies, we'd probably all pay good money to sit in the classrooms of these gifted little teachers.

Babies today seem to have awareness of their surroundings at an astonishingly early age, and even empathy.

Why does it seem like the current crop of babies has taken some sort of gigantic developmental leap forward? Perhaps one explanation for this phenomenon is that we've become more aware of mothers' and infants' needs while the baby is in utero, especially concerning nutrition, and mothers are making different, and healthier, choices. But is that the only explanation? Because we spend so much time around babies in the work we do with parents and families, we've been asking this question often over the last several years, watching little ones and listening to story after story from their parents, extended family, caregivers, pediatricians, and teachers. Doctors and nurses tell us that whereas babies in hospital nurseries used to sleep most of the time, now they seem much more alert from the get-go. Baby-group teachers report that babies in their classes seem to have awareness of both their surroundings and other babies at an astonishingly early age, and even empathy; they've watched as one baby crawls to another who is crying to keep her company, offer a kiss, or even reach out and touch her cheek. In our own interactions with children, we've seen newborns track people across the room at only days old, one- and two-month-olds respond to their names, and babies not even six months old able to roll a ball back and forth, say "mama," or follow a parent's guidance to pet the kitty gently. At only a year and a half, Derek's granddaughter, Alexa, began to go into quiet meditation spontaneously during a typical afternoon's play!

As remarkable as the babies being born these days are, though, you've likely discovered that being the parent of a little bright light is not always easy. As the mother of this wide-awake child, you have no choice but to try to keep up with her. Unfortunately, that may mean that you're up in the wee, small hours counting sheep together, as your little one may fight sleep with unbelievable gusto. It may also mean that you worry a lot. If she doesn't like to eat, how will she gain weight? If she doesn't sleep, won't that affect her brain development? She may get bored easily, never stop moving, react to any slight change in her environment, chatter away all day long, and want to engage you constantly. Being this little person's mom can feel like a fun-filled amusement-park ride, but it can also be very stressful!

The Stresses of Parenting Today

Stress has always been part of the job description as a parent, and probably always will be. But the kind of stress a mom experiences these days, which has a lot to do with her confusion or confidence about what's best for her child, is different from that of previous generations largely because of her social isolation. In Western society particularly, lots of new moms don't live near their families of origin, as their mothers and grandmothers may have, and it's more difficult to impart time-tested wisdom handed down from grandmom to mom, or from aunties, older siblings, cousins, and other extended family, when physical distance prevents frequent communication. (Phone, e-mail, and video chat will never replace a live body standing next to you to help troubleshoot a crying baby, or at least take a turn holding her.) The quality of a mom's relationship with her own mom and extended family matters a lot, too; where there is emotional disconnect due to unresolved conflict, a new mom won't be as open to input and advice, no matter how sound it is, and it may not even be forthcoming. A mom's sense of social support is further impacted by the availability and accessibility of resources like mom-and-baby classes, and she may not have as much time for friendships post-baby or as much in common with friends who aren't moms. On top of everything else, having a new baby can wreak havoc on even the most stable couple relationship and can cause new concerns about finances, work, and physical health and well-being, too.

The trickle-down effect of parental stress on children has been making lots of headlines in recent times. According to one study, for example, parents' stress directly impacts a child's propensity to become ill, and it may impact her developing immune system as well.[1] Another study found that parental stress in early childhood affected DNA methylation, a biochemical process that alters genetic expression, in later childhood.[2] In a survey by the American Psychological Association, 86 percent of children reported that their parents' stress caused them to feel negative emotions such as sadness, worry, or frustration, despite the fact that more than two-thirds of their parents reported that their stress had no impact on their child.[3] Equally alarming is the adverse effect that long-term stress can have on a child's brain development and overall well-being. According to the Centers for Disease Control and Prevention, "toxic stress," in which elevated levels of stress hormones like cortisol and adrenaline are present in a child's body for a prolonged time, has been shown to impact children in the following ways:[4]

- Toxic stress can impair the connection of brain circuits and lead to the development of a smaller brain.

- Children can become overly reactive to adverse experiences throughout their lives, developing a low stress threshold.

- High levels of stress hormones can suppress the body's immune response, leading to chronic health problems.

- Sustained high levels of certain stress hormones can damage areas of the brain important for learning and memory.

So because your baby is so strongly attuned to everything in her environment, and most especially to you, the stakes are high. When it comes to stress—and everything else, for that matter—there are no hiding places. To a sensitive, highly aware child, you are basically transparent. The pressure from your job, your financial woes, the pent-up resentment toward your mother, your negative feelings about your body, the simmering tension in your marriage—your child picks up on every bit of it. How? From the tone of your voice, your overall mood, the rhythm of your body movements, how you're moving your eyes, and the way you're interacting with your significant other—in other words, she learns about you by being with you. In fact, because she's *so* tuned in, she may be even more aware than you are of what you're feeling. Everything in your baby's environment is up for grabs as far as she is concerned, and because she's so keen on taking it all in, grab she will.

The reflection of your thoughts, mood, and behavior will show up with laserlike precision in the mirror image of your child.

What About Papas?

Dads and babies are strongly connected, too, of course. This book is geared toward mamas because moms are often the primary caretakers, and because the mother-baby connection is unique given that the baby spends forty weeks in mom's belly before arriving into the world. But there are lots of important ways that a dad's energy affects the baby, too, as well as the couple relationship—and we'll be addressing both of these subjects, and plenty more, in an upcoming book especially for you.

So what does all of this mean on a practical, day-to-day level for you and your baby? In a nutshell, the reflection of your thoughts, mood, and behavior will often show up with laserlike precision in the mirror image of your child. Here's an example: your mother calls, and after a few minutes you make an excuse to get off the phone; she's been driving you crazy, questioning your decisions and offering nonstop advice since the baby was born. Minutes later, your baby has a meltdown of monumental proportions. Coincidence? Maybe. Or maybe your child is quite literally acting out the anger you feel at your mother for the way she criticizes you all the time, which you tend to push down but rose a bit closer to the surface when she called.

Does that sound far-fetched? The truth is that you actually did the same thing as a child yourself, though of course you didn't realize what you were doing. It's what all children do. The idea that kids are mirroring back the consciousness of their parents is actually nothing new; it's just that because the children being born these days seem so highly attuned to their environment, their reflection of mom and dad's mood, emotions, and actions seems to appear very quickly and vividly. Even when you're not aware of it, your stress and negativity have an immediate, and potentially lasting, effect on your child's mood and behavior. Stress manifests in children similarly to how it manifests in adults, and its effects may include everything from indigestion and poor sleep to crying, fussy moods, and, when older, their own stress and anxiety. A baby who's happy and resilient today, if exposed to chronic stress, may seem like a different child in a few short years.

> Even when you're not aware of it, your stress and negativity have an immediate, and potentially lasting, effect on your child's mood and behavior.

Now, before you have a panic attack—the last thing an already overwhelmed parent needs is one more thing to worry about—let's get real: No one is perfect, and there's not a parent alive who doesn't have emotional and psychological baggage and plenty of stress. Being the parent of a highly attuned child, though, may motivate you to take a closer look at some of those crumbs you may be sweeping under the rug, because what you push down, hide, deny, and ignore will inevitably come back to visit you in the form of the adorable little mirror in front of you. What's more, that habit of avoidance, ironically, is largely what's *causing* your stress—and probably stems all the way back to your own childhood. Here's why: *You* were once a very attuned, aware little being who arrived in your parents' arms, delighting and alarming them by how alert *you* seemed. But no matter how loving and well-intentioned your parents were, they most likely didn't know how to recognize or appreciate your high level of sensory perception. It simply didn't occur to them to say, "Let me show you how to use that sensory acuity to your advantage, so you can stay balanced and use the information you're picking up on to understand yourself and the world." Instead, you got messages that certain emotions or behaviors weren't welcome in your home or out in the world, so you found ways to slow down or even block what you were feeling. In other words, you did your best to tuck those parts of yourself away into neat little boxes to survive and to "fit in"—and that's where the anxiety began. Anxiety is the result of hiding parts of ourselves that we don't want other people to see, and the more and the longer we do that, the more anxiety—and stress—we feel.

Today, as an adult, you may have found some healthy ways to manage your stress; maybe you do yoga or meditate, or maybe you walk, go to the gym, cook, garden, or paint. Or should we say, maybe you *used* to do those things before you became a mom! On the other hand, maybe you deal with stress in some not-so-healthy ways, such as with food, alcohol, or shopping; you may also be quite masterful at hiding it. If you fall into the latter camp, there are probably very few, if any, who know the inner turmoil that goes on inside of you much if not most of the time. The stressed-out mamas we've talked with over the years have described an ongoing thought-loop that spews a litany of potential worries: the slightly too familiar relationship your husband has with a coworker, the upcoming family gathering with the snarky sister-in-law who always tries to one-up you, the question of whether you're stimulating the baby enough to promote healthy brain development, the seesaw between craving balance as a mom and giving that idea the proverbial finger because it seems so unattainable. As two people who talk with lots of moms, we promise you that you are not the only one who thinks about these things!

The Effects of Stress

Not all stress is bad; when we're in a state of high alert, the brain releases stress hormones that give us energy to attend to the situation at hand, and that extra boost of energy can come in handy for a mom at times. When we carry ongoing stress, though, we also have chronically elevated levels of stress hormones, which can cause us to gain weight, weaken our immune system, and lead to other physical and mental health problems.

So you've brought a little bright light into the world, and perhaps part of what she is here to do is to help you find a new perspective. Maybe she's here to show you how being in touch with your emotions and sensory perception, which connect directly to your intuition, or mama instincts, is actually not a liability at all but an asset that can help you make choices and decisions that serve both you and your baby very well. Maybe your wide-awake child is here to help you open your own eyes to some of that heavy baggage you carry around—those habits of stress, negativity, and worry, for instance—which is weighing you down and preventing you from having the kind of life experience you really want to have. As bright as she is, though, your child still very much needs you to be her parent; she's looking to you to set the tone and the pace in the relationship, and she'll take whatever you've got. By becoming more aware of that reflection that she's mirroring back, you can learn to share your strengths rather than your challenges.

So if you want to be the best parent you can be to this extraordinary but sometimes demanding child, it seems clear that you're going to need a game plan. There are loads of books out there that talk about how to parent your child, but what about what *you* need as the parent? Let's start here: What would it be like to feel completely empowered regardless of whatever is going on around you or what your baby is doing, and so clear and confident in your parenting choices that you never doubted yourself at all? Okay, how about feeling that way *most* of the time? We wholeheartedly believe that this is not only possible but that you already have all you need to achieve it. Whether you had a child weeks or months ago, or whether you're well past the infancy stage by now, you have a vast library of parenting resources and wisdom lying within you just waiting to be tapped. Hopefully you've already made this discovery on your own, though you may feel baffled about why some days you feel like a rock star—parenting and taking care of your child with a spirit of verve, energy, and wit—whereas other days you can't even get a ticket to the show. Here's the secret: your parenting mojo flows strongly when you're calm and centered but slows to a trickle when you're stressed.

> Your parenting mojo flows strongly when you're calm and centered but slows to a trickle when you're stressed.

When we say "calm and centered," we are *not* talking about the kind of fake calm that comes from pretending everything is always okay (that isn't really calm but rather denial and suppression, which causes—you guessed it—stress), nor are we suggesting that you become some kind of Zen robot who has no feelings and no personality. We once saw a funny cartoon in the *New Yorker* with a mom and child holding hands; the caption read, *Mommy needs to get mad at you in a weird calm voice now*. That's no way to live! What we're talking about instead is being proactive about managing your energy so you can be proactive about what you share with your child. How do you go about managing your energy? By getting out of your head and into your body, feeling your feelings instead of avoiding them, and focusing more on the connection between you and your baby than on "doing it right" as a mom. It's really that simple.

When you take responsibility for managing your energy rather than allowing your thoughts, your emotions, other people, or life circumstances to manage you, you share your best self with the baby, your husband or partner, your parents and in-laws, and everyone else in your orbit. It's not about pretending to feel thrilled that your baby is up again at night or happy when you're experiencing inexplicable sadness as a new mom; on the contrary, it's about *acknowledging* that you're frustrated, sad, or anxious, and then allowing those feelings to express. It's your *unacknowledged* emotions that bounce around your household, unclaimed, for your baby to pick up on; once acknowledged, their impact diminishes considerably.

When you take responsibility for managing your energy rather than allowing your thoughts, your emotions, other people, or life circumstances to manage you, you share your best self with the baby.

Choosing to embrace your experience as a mom rather than resisting it allows you to be exactly who and what you are: happy and sad, ugly and beautiful, kind and bitchy, loving life and hating it, adoring of your child and also wishing, at times, that the stork would take her back up to the big baby nest in the sky for a few hours so you could finally get some rest. It's really okay to feel *all* of those things, and you may sometimes feel them all within a span of ten minutes! When you welcome and accept whatever you are experiencing, you not only feel more calm and balanced, you feel much better equipped to make clear decisions as a mom, too; you seem to know, instinctively, the right thing to do, or at the very least you have the courage to take a leap of faith and give it your best shot, knowing that no matter what, you'll learn something valuable that will make you an even better parent. Who you are affects your baby much more powerfully than what you do; she is like a little tuning fork, vibrating at the same tone you are offering.

Who you are affects your baby much more powerfully than what you do.

So where does all of this leave you, a busy, tired, often overwhelmed mom who is pumping like a madwoman to keep up your milk supply, trying to remember how long the pureed sweet potatoes have been in the fridge, doing the laundry, driving to appointments, singing "Itsy Bitsy Spider" for the umpteenth time, and trolling the Internet for the latest on the baby pain reliever recall—not to mention tending to your *paid* job and acknowledging your spouse once in a while? Squarely in the driver's seat, actually, because you can empower yourself in any moment by making a choice: to avoid what's going on inside of you, which causes stress, or to welcome the truth of your experience, and the sense of calm that results—which you can then share with your child. You know the saying "When Mama ain't happy, ain't nobody happy"? Well, the flip side is also true: when Mama is happy, everyone else is happier, too—and especially your child! Strong will, big personality and all, your child takes her cues for how to think, feel, and act from you. When you live in your own center, you teach your child how to live in her center, too.

The Brain, Fear, and Safety

Whether you decide to react with fear and emotion to a situation or to respond more calmly has a lot to do with which part of your brain is in charge. The brain can be divided into three main parts:

- The primitive brain, which is responsible for basic functions like heart rate and breathing.

- The emotional brain, or limbic system, which helps regulate emotions and also has a powerful influence on memory.

- The rational brain, or neocortex, which is responsible for things like logical thinking and impulse control.

One part of the brain called the *amygdala*, located within the limbic system, plays a very specific role: to be on the lookout for danger. It is constantly asking, "Is it safe?" If there are no perceived threats, you feel calm, and the neocortex can help you respond to sensory input in a balanced way, with logic and reason. But when the amygdala senses danger, it acts like there's a five-alarm fire, and our rational mind can be bypassed.

Once the amygdala decides that there's a threat to your safety, the sympathetic nervous system sends stress hormones like adrenaline and cortisol into your body, triggering a reaction known as "fight, flight, or freeze."

- Fight reactions include blaming, criticizing, arguing, and aggression.

- Flight reactions include leaving the environment, avoiding, ignoring, denying, and dismissing.

- Freeze reactions include shutting down emotions and feeling overwhelmed.

After the chemicals associated with strong emotion such as anger or fear are released into your body, it takes about ninety seconds for them to be completely reabsorbed so you feel calm again—unless you continue to think negative thoughts that amplify the emotion even further, in which case it can take much longer. Most of us aren't aware that our thoughts influence our feelings about an experience we've had, but this is good news; we can't control the immediate reactions we have to a situation, but we can control what happens next. That puts us in a very empow-ered place, as we can proactively manage our mood and overall state.

When the amygdala triggers a fight-flight-freeze reaction, you can signal to your brain that there is no real threat by:

- monitoring your thoughts about the situation at hand,

- paying attention to the emotions and physical sensa-tions in your body without getting swept up by them, and

- breathing deeply as you do each of these.

This will invoke the parasympathetic nervous system's counterbalancing effect to fight-flight-freeze, helping you to relax. We'll go into more detail about this process in Chapter 3, Connecting to Calm.

While science has made some interesting discoveries about the brain, our understanding of the brain and its functions are still very much a work in progress. Throughout this book, we'll share some very basic neuroscience to reinforce some of the ideas we present. While we are not neuroscientists, we offer this information to help make complex concepts more understandable.

The **Invisible** Umbilical

What no one tells you about having a child is that there are actually two births that occur. In addition to the birth of the physical baby, which is a monumental event all by itself, there is another very important experience that happens for every mother: the rebirth, or reawakening, of the past.

The Birth, and the Rebirth

When you become a mom, the baby in your arms engages you on every level: Physically, emotionally, and mentally, you become completely attuned to this little person and to all of her needs. This is nature's way of ensuring the baby's survival, and it's also the beginning of an extraordinary and very intimate new connection that you will both nurture, and that will nurture you both, for the rest of your lives. At the same time, the baby in front of you cannot help but also serve as a powerful connection back in time to yourself as a child, as well as to all of your earliest experiences. Through your interactions with your baby, memories of your own childhood and how you were parented yourself suddenly come flooding back, causing you to examine, or reexamine, some of the choices and decisions your own parents made and how those affected you. Part of the joy you experience when holding your baby and gazing into her eyes is remembering the miracle of your own arrival on the planet many years prior, and the innocence with which you began your own life. If you have memories of feeling loved and well cared for by your parents, you'll likely have a resurgence of those feelings now with your own baby, too. At the same time, though, whatever painful experiences you may have had as a child—times when you felt alone, ignored, rejected and *un*loved, for instance—are back to revisit you as well, and that often comes as quite a shock. Old childhood wounds you may have thought you had dealt with or tucked away into a neat, tidy little box are now unquestionably out of the box. *Way* out. This is justifiable cause for alarm.

Moms often experience this emotional intensity more strongly than dads do because moms are usually the baby's primary caregiver, meaning that in addition to dealing with hormonal surges, the volume is turned up on both the caretaking of the physical baby and the reintroduction to the past. Not only do you have this little being in front

> Through your interactions with your baby, memories of your own childhood and how you were parented suddenly come flooding back.

of you who requires feeding, changing, and care around the clock, but in every moment that you engage with her, that baby is also bringing back to life your own childhood joys, wounds, and positive and negative experiences. Some of this you may be aware of on a conscious level, but much of it will rekindle on an unconscious level, as you'll be quite busy tending to the child you've just welcomed, trying to figure out the best positions for feeding, researching burping techniques, and inventing clever tricks for getting her to sleep.

No wonder you feel thrown for such a loop!

The internal experience you have as a new mother is affected by the outward experience you are having, of course—if there are medical issues or if a baby is colicky, for instance, it's understandable that you would feel worry or stress—but a lot of what goes on inside of a new mom has to do with these doors that are opening to the past. You may function well enough on the outside as the tired-but-doting new parent who tries to laugh at herself as she finds her way. Privately, though, you may wonder why you sometimes feel overwhelmed by your baby's needs, and you may mistakenly believe that there is something wrong with you for feeling this way. It's a terrible position to be in as a mother; mom, so we are led to believe, is supposed to rise above it all, steering the ship through any storm and stretching her love and comfort like soft angel wings around the child who desperately needs her protection. At times, though, you may feel like you just want to crawl under a rock.

> In every moment that you engage with the baby, she is bringing back to life your own childhood joys, wounds, and positive and negative experiences.

I'm Fine, Thank You

Some of you might be thinking, *You know, I'm doing okay as a new mom—I have my moments, but I feel like I'm managing my stress pretty darn well.* If so, good for you! Just be aware, though, that you may actually have some stress that's manifesting in subtle ways that aren't readily apparent. These might include:

- Holding your breath when the baby cries

- Carrying tension in certain muscle groups, such as shoulders and neck

- Snapping at your husband or partner, or criticizing him

- Criticizing your own choices and decisions as a mom

- Feeling emotionally "flat"—neither happy nor sad, nor much of anything at all

- Using lots of sarcasm when you talk about your experiences as a mom (which can mask buried resentment)

- Feeling calm with your baby but emotionally triggered by an older child, if you're a mom to more than one

Whether you're feeling a little stressed as a new mom or a lot, the ideas and supports in this book can help you to feel like you're being the best mom you can to your baby.

How Your Baby's Brain Gets "Programmed"

At the same time that some of your past experiences are being reawakened as you parent your baby, another extraordinary phenomenon is happening, too; your baby is learning how to think, feel, and behave, and you are one of her most important teachers. Her survival instincts cause her to want to be like you, so she is paying close attention. Even when it seems like she's just being a baby—grabbing at your hair while nursing, laughing in delight as you tickle and squeeze her—your little bright light is actually studying you quite intensely, taking note of your tone of voice, your facial expressions, the way your touch feels, and all kinds of other sensory cues, in addition to how it generally feels to be around you. As mama—the one who carried her for (give or take) forty weeks and the person she's likely spending most of her time with—you are an indisputable star in the riveting reality show she calls life.

> Your baby's survival instincts cause her to want to be like you, so she is paying close attention.

As you may already know, your influence on your baby's experience started early. Science and the fields of fetal psychology and epigenetics, which studies genetic expression, can now show us that your baby began tuning into you when she was still in the womb. During your pregnancy, while the umbilical cord passed along nutrients from your body to your growing baby, she also picked up on your mood, your emotions, even your conversations—and your stress.[5] When the baby was born, she went right on tuning into mommy, using her five senses to imprint on your scent, your voice, the taste of your milk, and the feeling of your arms around her. But her attunement didn't stop there. Just as she did in utero, she's continued to pick up on your mood and emotions, too, and new research indicates just how powerfully contagious these can be. Emerging science on mirror neurons, for example, suggests that when your baby recognizes emotion in your facial expressions, she can feel what you're feeling. Other research has documented the powerful influence of a baby's early social interactions on both her current and future behavior.[6]

So even though the physical umbilical cord was cut at birth, it's as though there's an *invisible* umbilical that continues to connect the two of you at all times. Remember how much your parents' mental and emotional states affected you when you were a child yourself? Maybe you had a mother who was depressed much of the time or who always worried that something bad was going to happen; maybe your father had an explosive temper or always seemed stressed about money. Whatever the case, by now you've probably realized, at least to some extent, which of your parents' habits of thinking, feeling, and behaving rubbed off on you and eventually became your own.

Perceiving the World Through Feelings

Scientists like neurologist Jill Bolte Taylor, author of *My Stroke of Insight*, tell us that preverbal babies perceive the world primarily from their right brain, which governs feeling, tone of voice, and body language; in other words, what they're reading primarily is a parent's energy.[7] Even adults who have plenty of language skills, she says, still respond to how something feels first and foremost. When emotions arise, says Bolte Taylor, pay attention to what's going on in your body. Take anger: you can choose to either *be* angry or to take a step back and notice what anger feels like in your body. When you're emotionally triggered, she says, it takes only 90 seconds for the chemicals that accompany that emotion to flush in and flush completely out again. If emotions last longer than this, it's because our thoughts are continuing to run the same emotional circuitry.

Just as happened in your household growing up, now that you are the parent, your particular patterns of thinking, feeling, and behaving are influencing your child, too, as chronic, similar experiences of interacting with you light up the same neural pathways in her brain over and over. This is how the brain becomes "wired," or programmed in a particular way and how we develop tendencies toward positive or negative thoughts and feelings. Children are pretty well programmed by age five; the rest of their life experience—their degree of self-esteem and empathy, their emotional makeup, the quality of their relationships, their ability to accomplish goals and manage the stress of life's ups and downs—will be determined largely by what happens from birth until this age. This is why what you offer as a parent matters so much in these early years.

Children are pretty well programmed by age five; the rest of their life experienced is determined largely by what happens in these early years.

Consider this scenario:

Since the beginning, breastfeeding has been challenging for Melinda and her two-month-old baby, Henry. Melinda had always imagined that feeding would come naturally and easily, but Henry has had trouble latching on. Melinda has done her best to help Henry feed better—trying different positions and latch techniques, using nipple shields—and though Henry still struggles a bit, he is starting to gain more weight. But Melinda still feels lots of anxiety when Henry is feeding, and she beats herself up, feeling like she is letting him down. Unfortunately, nursing Henry makes Melinda feel over-the-top stressed, and she and the baby often both end up in tears.

Because Melinda is being hard on herself despite Henry's progress, she likely has a habit of self-criticism that stems all the way back to her own childhood; the seeds of that habit were probably planted by a parent who regularly criticized *her*, or perhaps often criticized themselves in her presence. In the scenario above, it might seem understandable that Henry's difficulty with feeding would be causing Melinda's stress, but doesn't it seem equally plausible that Melinda's stress and self-blame could be contributing to Henry's challenges? What's more, Melinda's habits of high anxiety during stress, and self-deprecation, could eventually become Henry's own.

In the mid-1990s, researchers proved the assertions of scientist Edward Lorenz, who suggested in the 1960s that a butterfly flapping its wings in one part of the world could affect weather patterns in another. So if a butterfly in Nebraska can affect the weather in China, it might seem easier to believe that your thoughts, feelings, and actions could have a powerful effect on your baby. A single negative or stressful thought, or even several here or there, will not affect your child long

term; rather, it's the unconscious *patterns* of
chronic stress and negativity that will pass
along to the baby via the invisible umbilical. If you are becoming aware of some
of your patterns of stress as you read
these words, don't panic; you haven't irre-
versibly harmed your baby, as your interaction with her in the present moment carries
more weight than whatever happened in the past.

> it's the unconscious *patterns* of chronic stress and negativity that will pass along to the baby via the invisible umbilical.

It can be helpful to be aware of how you handle stress, though, so that
you have the option of making different choices going forward. In the
next chapter, we'll offer plenty of suggestions for how to do just that.

Understanding the Connection

Being aware of the invisible umbilical that connects you
and the baby, you might be wondering, *Whoa, am I never
off duty as a mom?* The answer is yes—and no. You have
every right to have some downtime without the baby, and to
have other interests, such as work and friendships, outside of
being a mom. At the same time, even when you're not physically with her, the baby is still connected to you energetically
and can sense whether you yourself are secure in being
apart from her physically or whether you feel guilty or worried
about leaving. Understanding that this connection exists can
help motivate you to monitor negative thoughts and feelings and to create a healthy, balanced relationship with your
baby that makes room for both your needs and hers.

The Internal Movie Theater

Let's take a closer look at how our habits of thinking, feeling, and behaving are created. As a child grows, she is constantly creating impressions of her life experiences. These impressions are made up of input from her five senses, as well as what she senses internally through her intuition. She then ascribes meaning to her experiences by adding layers of her own thoughts and feelings to the original impressions. She can revisit, or remember, impressions of her most meaningful experiences anytime she wishes by replaying them like multisensory movies in a kind of internal home theater in her mind, and, if she has a riveting experience that brings up a lot of emotional charge, she'll likely watch the movie-memory of it again and again. This cinematic experience is endlessly fascinating and entertaining, what with all of the drama, action, romance, and comedy it serves up; some kids tend to pop in and out of their theater for quick fifteen-second shorts, whereas others spend so many hours there that their butt is permanently imprinted into the chair in front of the screen. You may remember your own tendencies toward one or the other when you were a child yourself.

Our Internal Theater

When we spend time with memories in our internal theater, each of us has a slightly different sensory experience. For some, the experience is largely visual; we see scenes from both recent and long-term memories being played out on a screen in our minds. For others, the experience is more auditory; we might listen to replays of conversations, or we might hear a voice in our head providing commentary and thoughts about experiences we've had. Some people experience memory mostly as feelings. Most of us have some combination of all three.

Now let's turn the spotlight on your baby, who has her own internal cinematic theater with a screen and a tiny chair (or maybe a swing). She doesn't visit it all that often yet because she hasn't had many experiences—nor does she much care to leave the present in order to visit the past and future, the way we do. At this age, she's more interested in the real-time movie in front of her. Here's an example: Let's say that your job causes you lots of stress. At the end of your long days, you're often tired and drained. Despite your best attempts to perk up for the baby when you're home in the evening, she picks up on your lack of eye contact, the tension in your voice and facial expression, and the jangly feeling she gets when you hold her; she also notices that when you're talking to her, you seem a bit distracted. She senses that something's bothering you, but she doesn't know what or why. Today, her reaction to your stress may be to cry and fuss and to generally seem out of sorts.

Over the next couple of years, though, your child will develop language. She'll become a very imaginative storyteller, creating some rather colorful distortions about her life experiences—some positive, some negative—and especially those in which she's interacting with you (as well as her other parent). Experiencing your stress at the end of the day at this point, and registering emotional disconnect, she might think, *Mommy doesn't seem very happy when she comes home. Maybe I'm doing something wrong to upset her.* That wouldn't be true, of course, but that's the way kids' minds work; when parents seem upset about something, children tend to make themselves the culprit. Her reaction to your stress now that she's older may be to talk back or act out behaviorally, and this will likely lead to some pretty charged interactions with you; maybe you'll find yourself yelling. This is around the time when her internal movie theater will begin to sell a lot more popcorn. Having repeated similar experiences with you, plus watching movies of those same scenes and reinforcing the powerful emotions she feels, she may start to make some pretty sweeping conclusions: *When I'm bad, Mommy doesn't love me.* This is how neural pathways deepen, and how we develop habits of thought and the fundamental belief systems that shape who we are and how we perceive ourselves, others, and the world. Neurons that fire together, wire together.

When parents seem upset about something, children tend to make themselves the culprit.

For better and worse, most of us continue to watch our childhood movies, and carry childhood beliefs, long after our childhood has passed. No one sends us a memo after we leave home saying, "Go ahead and clean out your cinematic library any old time now. You can trash the movie called *If I'm Quiet, I'll Be Loved* at age twenty-one, and by the time you're twenty-five, you can scuttle *I'm Not Allowed to Get Angry.* Hold on to *People Aren't Okay Unless I Take Care of Them* till you're about thirty, though, because you're going to be in a relationship with someone who's going to really enjoy holding hands while you watch that movie together." Now that you're a mom, some of these old movies may actually be in heavy rotation because your baby is reminding you of your own childhood. When a present experience reminds you of something in the past, what's happening is that your inner projectionist is queueing up movies of past events at the same time that similar events are unfolding in front of you today—often without your conscious awareness. If the movies that begin to play about the past are painful ones, the brain immediately registers danger, and you go into fight-flight-freeze. That's why your emotional reactions to certain scenarios with the baby feel so intense; you're both experiencing what's happening now and re-experiencing what happened in the past simultaneously.[8] Whether you react with stress or respond more calmly depends on which part of your brain is in charge; it's also largely a matter of habit. The good news is that habits can be changed.

The Benefits of
Staying Connected

As a mom, you've probably noticed by now that when you're calm, you feel connected to your baby and your instincts, and it's easier to make clear decisions about your baby's needs. When you're stressed, on the other hand, you feel disconnected from yourself and from your baby, too, and things can feel a lot more chaotic and confusing. When something stressful happens with the baby—you can't figure out what she needs, or she won't settle no matter what you do—it's sometimes easy to forget that staying nonreactive, and overriding fight-flight-freeze, is a *choice*. Whether you make that choice is not an evaluation of your parenting skills, but it's important to know that your choice affects not only you but your little bright light as well. When you disconnect from yourself during times of stress, you disconnect from your baby, too, and it becomes more challenging to respond to her needs accurately; what's more, because you are her teacher, she may eventually learn to disconnect from herself during stressful situations, just like you. As mom, you have an extraordinary ability to influence the kind of experiences your baby has and thus the way her brain is wired.[9] This will either feel like an amazing opportunity or a lot of pressure, depending on your menu of offerings.

As you're reading these words, whether you're thinking, *Help! I'm a new parent and I've never been so stressed in all my life* or, *I have my good moments and my less-than-good moments, but I wouldn't mind some more of the good ones,* you're in the right place. Whatever your experience of being a new mom, this book is designed to help you enjoy your parenting experience as much as possible so that you can share the best of what you have to offer with your baby. It's not about being perfect, nor is it about being positive all the time; you're allowed to lose it at times as a mom! Instead, it's about being authentic. As you bring more awareness and acceptance to your experiences, positive and negative, you'll leave fewer "leftovers" for the baby—or anyone else, for that matter—to pick up on. In any relationship—with a child, spouse, friend, or family member—we're at our best when we're able to show up fully for what's being exchanged. The more present we are, the more connected to each other we feel, and the more connected to each other we feel, the more that connection nurtures each of the people experiencing it. After her physical needs are met, there's arguably nothing more

> As you bring more awareness and acceptance to your experiences, positive and negative, you'll leave fewer "leftovers" for the baby to pick up on.

important you could offer your baby than your own well-being, as this will provide an inexhaustible wellspring from which you can offer her love and whatever else she needs.

So here's the paradox: parenting brings tremendous challenges, and also tremendous gifts. This beautiful miracle in a tiny package, otherwise known as your baby, is actually a very powerful teacher in a very clever, adorable disguise. She has come into your life not only to receive all of your love, nurturing, and guidance but also to inspire you to take a deeper look at your habits and choices. Your relationship with your baby can help you to stretch your capacity for love, joy, and fulfillment in all of your other relationships, too, including the one with yourself. Parenting a little bright light can be an intense but exhilarating experience; it comes with plenty of trial and tribulation, but it also brings loads of joy and celebration. In Chapter 3, we're going to offer some supports for finding and staying in your center as a mom—or at least spending more time there than you may currently be doing. This way, you'll feel more equipped to manage the ups and downs of daily life as a mom, you'll have clearer access to your mama instincts, and you'll bring more joy to your experience of being a mom. This is a foundation from which you and your baby can build a strong, loving connection—and thrive.

The Other (Ugly) Truth About Motherhood

There is a very common truth about parenting that many moms don't feel comfortable acknowledging: even though you love your baby, sometimes you don't enjoy being a mom. It's exhausting; the baby cries too much or sleeps too little, being with her brings up painful emotions at times, and it just feels hard. If you have ever entertained thoughts like these—and then felt engulfed by waves of guilt and shame—please know that you are far from alone; every mom we've talked to has similar sentiments now and then. Feeling this way doesn't mean you're a bad mom, it just means you get overwhelmed at times.

If you are having negative thoughts and feelings about being a mom on a regular basis that are affecting your ability to function or take care of your baby, though, you may have postpartum depression. Talk to a professional who can help determine whether treatment may be a good option for you.

CHAPTER 3

Connecting to Calm

As every mother knows, one of the most important things you can do for your child's well-being is to nurture a relationship based on healthy, secure attachment and a sense of trust. The cornerstone of healthy attachment is being able to attune to your baby and to accurately read and respond to her cues, communication, and signals often enough that you create a secure bond to nurture her physical, social, and emotional development. That's no small task for even a calm mama on a full night's sleep, and, if you've got some emotional inner turmoil that's been competing with your child for your energy and attention—and what mom doesn't?—you may have a hard time being fully present with her at times, and some guilt and anxiety about that to boot. This dynamic is not exactly a prescription for feeling calm and happy.

What's more, your little bright light is extremely attuned to you, meaning that your thoughts, feelings, and actions have a direct and immediate effect on her. As we said in Chapter 2, your stress and negativity unfortunately do pass right along to your baby through the invisible umbilical, but the flip side is also true: when you are calm and centered, you share those gifts with her as well. So how exactly do you stay centered, given that life as a mom has more ups and downs than, say, a sleepless baby? The good news is that being centered is *not* about trying to be positive and happy all the time; rather, it's about stepping all the way into whatever you are experiencing as a mom—the good, the bad, and the ugly—rather than judging or dismissing it. Stress lies in the discrepancy between what you believe you *should* feel and what you actually feel, between what you believe *should* be happening and what is actually happening, between who you believe you *should* be as a mom and who you actually are. Owning the truth of your experience as a mom, whatever it is, means that you're giving yourself permission to be you, not some supermom who has all the answers and never lets her baby—or anyone else—down. It also has the added benefit of helping you tap into your mama instincts, which are virtually impossible to access when you're stressed but flow much more easily when you're more relaxed.

> Stress lies in the discrepancy between what you believe you should feel and what you actually feel.

One of the key ingredients to feeling happy in any relationship is the willingness to bring 100 percent of yourself to the table, and the relationship with your baby is no exception. If you disconnect from yourself by denying or hiding parts of yourself or feelings you believe shouldn't be there, you disconnect from her, too. Can you imagine saying to your baby, "Honey, you can be happy anytime you want, but please don't ever be sad, angry, or scared"? Of course not! Though that might actually sound like a nice fantasy, hopefully you recognize how unhealthy that would be for her. And if that's true for her, isn't it also true for you? If you want your child to have the full freedom of self-expression you were likely not given as a child yourself, how will you be able to teach her that if you are not according yourself the same freedom? As the parent, your job is not to be an unwavering rock of strength for her but to show her what it is to be human; she needs to witness you having feelings so she knows what they are and how to allow them when she has them, too. We're not suggesting that you share with her all of your woes, as you *are* indeed the parent, but if you get into the practice of allowing your emotions to surface and welcoming them, you'll find that they rise up—even quite strongly at times—and then pass like the weather, just like they do for children, who haven't learned how to block them.

As you attune to yourself by tolerating your discomfort—which may seem difficult at times, thanks to those old movies from the past that are in heavy rotation as a new mom—you'll feel much better able to attune to your baby, too. You'll be more adept at recognizing the subtler aspects of her communication, and therefore better able to understand what she needs, because you're already practicing doing this with yourself. You might even find that you seem to know what she needs before she tells you! The guidance, resources, creativity, and wisdom you need to take care of your baby will seem to flow much more easily, from a kind of internal stream. When mom is relaxed, her baby thrives.

Finding Your Center

Some mamas seem calm and fairly confident about connecting with their internal guidance; others seem to feel more anxiety and may worry more. Your tendencies one way or the other have to do with your individual makeup, the way you were raised, and habit. If centering yourself—which we are defining as standing in the truth of your experience, right here, right now—doesn't come easily for you, the good news is that it's never too late to learn how. And if you consider yourself a fairly calm mama already, you can always benefit from deepening your practice of staying present with whatever is happening with you or your baby, even if it's uncomfortable.

The processes we offer in this chapter have worked well for many moms just as we've presented them here, though it's not important that you follow the steps in each exercise perfectly; please feel free to adapt them, change them, and use them in whatever way feels good to you. Play and have fun, and whatever you do, don't worry about doing it right! These supports are about helping you to remember that while you don't have a choice about what happens as a mom, you always have a choice about how you respond.

Last but not least, please feel free to use these tools not just as triage during a crisis but also preventively; there is absolutely no downside to feeling as centered and relaxed as possible at any point throughout your day. If anxiety or stress do start to spike up, whether because of something going on with your child or because of another stressful trigger, like a caregiver who called in sick or an argument with your spouse, try to get in the habit of reaching for one of these supports at the *first* sign of stress rather than once you're already pulling your hair out; that way, you can defuse stress much more quickly and easily. To get a sense of how much you're shifting with each one, use a number on a 1 to 10 scale to measure your level of stress before and after each process, with 10 being the most stressed.

Breath of Life

Breathing is arguably the most important thing we can do. It not only sustains our life, it also gives us energy, rids the body of toxins, and helps us manage stress. The funny thing is, though, hardly any of us know how to do it properly. But babies do. Did you ever notice that when your baby is lying on her back, her belly goes up and down as she breathes? That's because she's breathing with her diaphragm. Most adults breathe much more shallowly, not engaging their diaphragm much, if at all.

Lie on your back and place a medium-size book on your abdomen; the weight of the book will engage your diaphragm and remind you of what it feels like to breathe this way. (If you've given birth fairly recently, place your hands just below your rib cage and apply gentle pressure.) Now sit up comfortably, feet on the floor, and try this:

- As you begin to inhale, imagine that you are filling a balloon inside of your stomach with air.

- Then bring your breath up into your chest, gently inhaling to full capacity. Don't push further than what's comfortable.

- Hold for a beat; you'll likely feel your neck and shoulders, and other tense places in your body, relax a bit.

- Now exhale.

Follow this sequence as you breathe throughout the day. If it's helpful, you can count while inhaling and exhaling; for example, you can count to three while breathing in, then count backwards from three while breathing out. Taking a deep breath, or several, is the fastest, easiest way to bring yourself into the moment, wherever you are and whatever you are doing; it's like a calm and happy pill anytime you need it.

Taking a deep breath, or several, is the fastest, easiest way to bring yourself into the moment, wherever you are and whatever you are doing.

When your baby is fussy, try taking one to three deep breaths and watch what happens. When babies start to fuss in our Calm Mama, Happy Baby classes, we invite all of the moms to take three deep breaths together; time and again, the room gets so quiet and still that you can hear a pin drop. This is the most powerful illustration we've seen of a mom calming herself and then sharing that calm with the baby. Try it yourself! (To see a video demonstration of how to breathe properly, please visit our website, calmandhappy.com.)

Here are two variations on the breath that you can also use as needed.

Calming Breath (Moon Breath)

Use this one to begin calming as soon as you notice anxiety, tension, or frustration starting to kick in.

- Hold your right nostril with your thumb.

- Breathe in to a count of five; make sure to inhale so your upper chest fills with air.

- Exhale to a count of six; make sure to exhale so all the air leaves your abdomen.

- After a month or so of practice, you can slowly begin to increase both the inhale and the exhale counts longer. A longer exhale signals your brain to turn the volume down on your sympathetic nervous system (which governs fight-flight-freeze) and turn the volume up on your parasympathetic nervous system (which helps you to calm and relax).

Energizing Breath (Sun Breath)

Use this one to bring in more energy when you need a boost, or when you're feeling tired or lethargic.

- Hold your left nostril with your thumb.

- Breathe in to a count of five; make sure to inhale so your upper chest fills with air.

- Exhale to a count of six; make sure to exhale so all the air leaves your abdomen.

- After a month, you can slowly begin to increase the inhale and exhale counts longer.

CALM Mama

Use this process anytime, anywhere: when your baby is fussing, when she's getting frustrated trying to do something new (like roll or crawl), or when she's adjusting to a transition (like changing into PJs or stopping playtime for a nap). You can also work with these steps anytime throughout your day to feel as connected to yourself and your baby as possible. Note that the goal here is *not* to stop the baby from crying if she's upset, or to prevent either of you from experiencing whatever you are experiencing, but rather to remain as present as possible so you can attend to her with all of your resources. Sometimes babies just cry no matter how you try to help, and that's really okay, even though it's not always fun!

As you read through these steps, you might be wondering, *How the heck am I going to have time to do all of this when my baby is crying and needs me?* It might sound like we're asking you to do a lot before you attend to your little one, but we're just slowing things down so we can explain each of the steps clearly. When you're with your baby in the moment, you'll respond in a matter of seconds, and with just a little practice, that's about as long as this process will take.

You'll connect with *yourself* first, then your baby. Why wouldn't you just jump in and attend to the baby, especially if she's fussing? Well, you know when you're on an airplane, and you're asked to put the oxygen mask on yourself as the adult first, then help your child? It's the same in this scenario: if you aren't breathing—in other words, if you're checked out, shut down, tense, or anxious—you'll be reacting from a place of disconnection and fear, and you won't feel nearly as clear about how best to respond to the baby. What's more, because of the invisible umbilical, if you're stressed and anxious while you attend to her, you might inadvertently add to her distress.

We use the acronym CALM as a guide for remembering the steps, which are:

C: Cancel negative thoughts
A: Allow your feelings
L: Link up and listen
M: Mirror

C: Cancel Negative Thoughts

When we get stressed, we stop breathing properly. And when we stop breathing properly, we tend to check out of our bodies and go into our heads. Stress plus being in your head usually equals lots of negative thinking about all the things that are *wrong* in your world, which makes you even more stressed. The number one cause of stress for you as a mom is actually not the physical caretaking of the baby but the negative thoughts that loop repeatedly in your mind throughout the day about whatever is unfolding in front of you, whether the baby won't eat or sleep or the pediatrician has kept you waiting for nearly an hour. See if any of these thoughts sound familiar:

> The number one cause of stress for you as a mom is actually not the physical caretaking of the baby but the negative thoughts that loop repeatedly in your mind throughout the day.

- *The baby won't latch on—what am I doing wrong?*
- *My mother is so selfish. She only thinks about herself, not what I need as a new mom.*
- *I can't believe my brother has only come to see the baby once since she was born.*
- *This traffic is ridiculous. I'm going to be late for the doctor appointment.*
- *Why won't the baby nap? All the books said she should be napping three times a day, and she refuses!*

It's not that you're thrilled that the baby won't latch on or isn't napping, but dwelling on what's going wrong will only make you stressed and may prevent you from feeling clear about how best to help. So right now, take a deep breath in and just let all that negative thinking go out with your exhale breath. Feels better already, doesn't it?

A: Allow Your Feelings

Now bring your full awareness to your body. Feel your feet on the ground and take another big, deep breath. Then ask yourself, *What physical sensations or emotions am I feeling?* (If it's easier, keep it simple: anxiety, sadness, and anger are the primary emotions that will come up when you're stressed.) Now describe what you're experiencing with as much detail as possible:

- *Where in my body am I feeling this sensation or emotion?*
- *What does this feeling feel like?*
  - *Is it strong or faint?*
  - *Is it dull or sharp?*
  - *Is it heavy or light?*
  - *Is it moving or staying still?*
  - *Does it have a color or a shape?*

Describing what you're feeling in detail helps you stay present in your body. Whatever you are feeling, just notice; avoid any judgment or analysis of *why* you're feeling what you are, as that will take you out of your body and back into your head. Here are some examples of what you might discover:

- *I'm flippin' exhausted. It feels like I just ran a 10K marathon.*
- *I'm hungry. I actually forgot to each lunch.*
- *There's a dull, heavy pain in my left shoulder. It stretches up into my neck, too, and it's kind of throbbing.*

- *I feel sad. It's like a hollow, achy, burning feeling in my throat. Feels like there's a waterfall of tears right behind it.*

- *I'm feeling a lot of anxiety, mostly in my stomach. It's like a knot of tightness.*

- *My right wrist is stiff, and it really hurts to move it. There are sharp red spikes of pain shooting out.*

If it helps, you can even say these things out loud. "Naming and claiming" what you're feeling helps you stay present with it, regardless of whether the sensations you're feeling are comfortable or uncomfortable, pleasant or unpleasant. This is because you're accepting them rather than resisting, avoiding, or reacting, all of which are fear-based versions of fight-flight-freeze. *Breathe into the places where you feel tension or emotion,* and see if anything wants to soften a bit.

You Are the Projectionist

The stronger your anxiety, sadness, and anger in any moment, the more likely it is that the projectionist in your internal movie theater is playing an unpleasant scene or two from your past, even if you're not aware that that's happening. News flash: You don't have to keep watching that movie. By getting out of your head and into your body, you also come out of your internal movie theater and into the present moment.

L: Link Up and Listen

Now that you've connected with yourself by acknowledging whatever you are experiencing, connect with the baby by focusing on the invisible umbilical that links the two of you at all times. This channel allows you to share a back-and-forth flow of communication and information, and it allows for a nuanced read on the baby and her needs. As you connect with her, intend that you are sharing your love, and then tune in and gather information about what she is experiencing. Hold an attitude of curiosity—*I wonder what you're trying to tell me?*—rather than rushing to "fix" the baby's upset, which has fear attached to it. Pay attention as you listen to your five senses and your sixth sense, or intuition, too:

- If she's crying, what does that *sound* like? Is it a loud, piercing wail or mild fussing? Does it sound like an urgent call for help or more like discomfort?

- What does she *look* like? Is her skin tone close to its normal color, or more pale or red? Is her face relaxed or all scrunched up? Are her eyes open or closed? Are her body movements fluid or disjointed?

- If you're holding her, what does she *feel* like? Is she hot or cool? Damp or dry? Squirmy or still?

- Are there any *smells* to be aware of—such as a good ol' poopy or gas?

- Is there anything that you *sense* internally—perhaps that she's overstimulated or needs a change of environment, or that she's ready to sleep or feed even if it isn't "time" yet?

As you attune to her, continue to check in with your own body sensations, too. What you are feeling is a source of valuable information for you. It's your attunement to the baby, and yourself, that will help you tap into your mama instincts and bring clarity about how best to attend to her.

M: Mirror

To let her know that you're listening and hearing her, use your words, tone of voice, touch, and facial expression to reflect whatever you're noticing:

- "You're so upset right now! Mom is listening to everything that you're saying."

- "You seem really warm, honey. I wonder if you're uncomfortable in that sweater?"

- "You were trying to roll, and your arm got stuck. You didn't like that."

- "Your eyes look red. I'll bet you're ready for a nap."

- "I'm not really sure what you need, sweetie, but I'm right here with you, and we're going to go through this together."

Mirroring is simply reflecting back to the baby what you've picked up using your senses, with empathy. Connecting with the baby this way helps her to "feel felt" and lets her know she's not alone in her experience.[10] Pay attention to how she's responding, following her lead and continuing to make adjustments as you read her. As you tune into your body, you'll know when to engage and when to back off a bit, like the rhythm of a dance. As your baby experiences you experiencing her in a calm way, she may begin to relax, too. How wonderful!

Mirroring Back

When a baby is crying, it can be tempting to try to soothe her by saying, "Don't cry!" or "You're okay!" That response, though, is actually a misattunement. If the baby is crying, she is clearly not okay! Don't be afraid of your baby's discomfort. Rather than glossing over her upset, try simply mirroring back to her whatever you are noticing. "Something is really bothering you" or, "That loud noise really surprised you!" might be a more accurate reflection of her experience.

After you've gone through the steps for CALM (remember that with practice, this will take only seconds), if the baby needs your assistance, by all means take action. Do whatever feels right—offer the breast or bottle; hold her or swaddle her; put her in her carrier, walk around the room, or go outside. Or maybe you'll feel like simply placing a hand on the baby's chest and holding a steady gaze with her, offering your love and presence without saying anything at all. Trust your mama instincts, and don't be afraid to experiment! If you're still unsure about what to do, don't panic; just do your best to attend to her, and if you try something and the baby continues to fuss anyway, just keep cycling through the steps for CALM if they're helpful. This way, you'll be lovingly keeping her company regardless of what's she's experiencing, which teaches her how to begin managing her own ups and downs.

When the brain senses danger, it sends stress hormones into the body and triggers the sympathetic nervous system's fight-flight-freeze response. CALM signals to the brain that you are safe and all is well, which activates the parasympathetic nervous system and helps you relax. Each time you choose to tolerate sensations of physical and emotional discomfort rather than avoiding them or reacting, you rewire your brain's neural circuitry and help create a new habit.

What the CALM process does is put a big pause in between what's happening with the baby and your response to what's happening. In that pause, you are centering yourself by acknowledging your own experience so you can respond to the baby with more calm and clarity than stress or anxiety. *Important:* Whatever you decide to do, do it from a place of trust and faith in yourself as a mom who is gaining experience and learning more all the time, rather than with self-deprecation or worry that you'll somehow get it wrong. We've noticed over the years that the mamas who second-guess themselves are pretty darn stressed most of the time, as we'll talk more about later in this book—and perhaps not coincidentally, stressed-out mamas often tend to have fussier babies. When you *decide* to respond to your baby

> What the CALM process does is put a big pause in between what's happening with the baby and your response to what's happening.

from a place of confidence that you're doing your best, even if you're unsure about what the result will be, the baby feels safe knowing that you are doing what you can to meet her needs. The energy with which you respond matters *far more* than what you do.

CALM in a Nutshell

- **Cancel negative thoughts** that focus on the idea that whatever is happening is "wrong." Take a deep breath in and release any negativity as you exhale.

- **Allow your feelings.** Without judgment, just notice the physical sensations and any emotions that are present in your body, describing them with as much detail as possible. Take another deep breath into any areas where you are feeling tension or emotion.

- **Link up and listen.** Now connect with the baby via the invisible umbilical; share your love with her and gather information about what she is experiencing, using both your physical senses and your sixth sense, or mama instincts.

- **Mirror** back to the baby what you're noticing about her experience, rather than trying to "fix" her upset. This way, the baby experiences you experiencing her in a calm way, which helps her calm, too.

Go ahead and attend to the baby however you feel is best—pick her up, rock her, take a walk outside. Keeping her company with calm, grounded energy is more important than what you do.

Tuning In to Your Baby's Signals

Every baby has different sensory needs; that's why some babies love to be held and others prefer more downtime, or why some babies seem to think getting their diaper changed is the greatest thing that could ever happen whereas others find it a miserable experience. Get to know your baby's preferences by tuning in and paying attention to:

- **Changes in mood.** Do your baby's mood changes seem to coincide with changes in the environment, the time of day, or hunger or tiredness? For example, if your baby is often cranky in the late morning, see if she might be sending you signals—less eye contact, lower energy— just before her mood dips. If so, you may want to try a nap or a feed when you see these signs.

- **Reactions to her environment.** Your baby might get overstimulated by having too many people around or become upset about schedule changes. Knowing her needs can help you plan accordingly.

- **Differences in your baby's cries.** Try to notice the difference between the baby's hungry cry and her tired cry. Pay particular attention to the volume, pitch, and intensity of the cry, as well as your baby's body language and facial expressions. An arched back, a scrunched-up face, eyes tightly closed to shut out the light, fingers curled up into fists, rubbing eyes, and active or calmer movement are all cues about your baby's emotional and physical state.

• **Her sensory preferences.** Some babies like to be held constantly or enjoy touch with deep pressure; others prefer a softer touch. Note your baby's preferences for sound, including music and the tone of your voice, as well as for visual stimulation, including color.

Learning what it takes to read, soothe, and comfort your baby takes practice, but your skills of perception and awareness about her needs will sharpen with time. Note that babies born prematurely, or with medical conditions, may have an unusually sensitive nervous system.

When Emotions Feel Overwhelming

If you experienced trauma as a child—for example, physical, sexual, or emotional abuse—or an intensely painful experience, such as the death of a close family member or your parents' divorce, your emotions may feel particularly strong. If you don't feel safe or comfortable with the emotions that are coming up for you as a new mom, reach out to a professional who can help determine whether treatment might be right for you.

Anchoring Calm

The practice of neurolinguistic programming (NLP), which helps people use the brain's natural wiring and language to create behavioral change, offers tools for shifting old habits and patterns that no longer serve us. One tool that can be particularly useful for moms is called an *anchor*. Here's how it works.

We are constantly taking in stimulation from the world through our five senses; when something happens that is meaningful to us, our brain sets off a chain reaction of thoughts, feelings, and sometimes behaviors, all of which can then become "anchors" for that experience. For example, there are probably certain songs you hear on the radio that immediately bring up a particular feeling—sadness, joy, romantic love—because you were feeling that way the first time you heard the song play. Anchors are created all the time without our conscious awareness, but we can consciously create anchors to help give us a choice about how to respond to a particular situation.

Wouldn't it be handy to be able to tap into feelings of calm and confidence throughout your day as a busy mom? Here are the steps for creating an anchor you can use any time you wish.

- Close your eyes and remember a time when you felt both calm and confident. It could be since becoming a mom, or it might be before you had a baby.

- Make sure that in the memory you are replaying in your internal theater, you are feeling *very* calm and *very* confident, as close to 10 on a 1 to 10 scale as you can get, with 10 being the most calm and confident. Bring to life vividly the details about where you are and what you are doing, seeing, hearing, and feeling.

- When you're as close as you can get to a 10, touch your left index finger to the middle knuckle on your right hand and hold it there for about fifteen seconds. Now you have an "anchor" for feeling calm and confident.

- When stress, irritation, or anxiety spike up throughout your day, you can acknowledge those feelings and then use your anchor to return to feeling more calm. You might even find that using your anchor helps your baby to calm, too.

- To reinforce your anchor, whenever you are feeling calm and confident throughout your day, or perhaps after following the steps for CALM or another exercise in this chapter, touch your index finger to your knuckle in the same way. The more often you reinforce your anchor, the more powerful it becomes; neurons that wire together, fire together.

You can also create anchors for feeling anything else you wish, such as strongly attuned to your baby, clear about your mama instincts, or alert and energetic.

Anchoring Baby's Calm

You can use anchors to help reinforce your baby's calm, too. You're probably already doing this without being aware of it; singing "Twinkle, Twinkle Little Star" is one example. Here's how to create an anchor for the baby.

- When your baby is calm and happy, gently stroke her ear, squeeze her leg, or stroke her cheek. These are just ideas; you can create the anchor in whatever way feels right to you.

- Reinforce your touch with language: "Mama sees that you're feeling so calm and happy right now!"

- When the baby is having difficulty settling, acknowledge what she's feeling, then use her anchor to help her calm—and maybe your own, too.

You're a Mirror

A baby's ability to self-regulate, or maintain an internal state of balance, is absolutely dependent on relationship. Silvan Tomkins, an early researcher who studied attachment, suggested that when a parent stays connected to her child while she experiences negative emotions, she helps that child to both reduce stress and increase her tolerance for stressful experiences in the future. A mother's ability to regulate *herself*, Tomkins found, strongly impacts her ability to create secure attachment in her child.[11] What's more, when you calm and regulate yourself, the baby learns how to regulate herself, too. Watching you take a deep breath, for example, activates her mirror neurons, which enable her to mirror your actions in her own mind as if she had performed them herself. V. S. Ramachandran, a pioneer in mirror neuron research, calls mirror neurons "empathy neurons" or "Dalai Lama neurons," as they are "dissolving the barrier between self and others."[12]

Tuning In Within

Do not underestimate the amount of information you can learn about your baby by getting still and tuning in.

You are the number one expert on your own baby, and you have a treasure trove of parenting wisdom inside of you—though you may not be accessing this wisdom as fully or as often as you could be. Do not underestimate the amount of information you can learn about your baby by getting still and tuning in. You'll need a few minutes of uninterrupted time for each of these exercises.

Accessing Clear Guidance

Use this exercise to tap into guidance for anything you'd like to have more clarity about as a mom, such as how to help your baby sleep better.

- Sitting comfortably, take three deep breaths. Close your eyes on the third exhale breath.

- Whatever it is you'd like guidance about, frame it as a clear question: for example, *How can I help the baby sleep better at night?* (Note: it's generally best to ask one question at a time, then wait for answers.)

- Now tune in and listen; stay open to whatever comes. You might hear words, you might get an idea, you might see a picture, you might get a feeling or just a sense of knowing— whatever kind of guidance comes is perfect for you. No need to analyze or evaluate the guidance you get in this step, just let the ideas come. And don't panic if nothing happens; answers to your question may pop up hours or even days later, while you're scrubbing the shower, changing a diaper, or talking to a mom friend. If you haven't had much experience accessing your guidance this way, it may take some practice to feel clear about the answers to your questions.

- If you'd like, keep pen and paper nearby to jot down notes, or record ideas into your phone.

You can also use your anchor for feeling calm and confident at the beginning of this exercise, and/or create an additional anchor afterward, when you're feeling strongly connected to clear inner guidance.

Trying It On

When you have an either-or choice to make about your baby's well-being—such as choosing to start solid foods with grains or veggies, or whether to hire one caregiver or another—and the answer doesn't seem clear, follow these steps to "try on" the choice before you decide.

- Sitting comfortably, take a deep breath and close your eyes.

- Imagine yourself making one of the choices, such as hiring one of the caregivers, and call up as much sensory detail as possible. See and hear yourself greeting this person as she comes to your house in the morning; imagine her playing with and holding the baby, and imagine what it feels like to leave the baby with this person as you go out to do errands. Feel, see, and hear as much detail as possible, and notice what happens in your body. Do you feel relaxed and open, or tense and tight?

- Now imagine making the other choice, in this case hiring the other caregiver, and check in again.

- What did making each choice feel like when you tried it on? When a choice feels right, you'll likely notice that your body feels expansive—your chest opens up, you feel relaxed, and you may get an excited, tingly feeling in your stomach as you feel anticipation. When something doesn't feel right, you'll likely have a restricted feeling in your body—your breathing may get shallower, your muscles may feel tight, and you might have a "sinking" feeling in your stomach.

To get a true read on what "yes" and "no" feel like in your body, you can "try on" something you already know to be right or not right for your baby, such as using one kind of swaddle or another. Experiment and see what you discover!

Baby OM

Babies naturally respond to the sound of OM, which is one interpretation of the sound they hear while in utero. It's also the sound that the universe makes, as NASA has recorded (and as the yogis in India have known for thousands of years). The sound of OM can help both you and your baby to calm, and you may find that it becomes an anchor for both of you.

- Place the baby on her back on a blanket on the floor, with you sitting in front of her.

- Take a deep breath in, and as you're exhaling make the sound OMMMMM. Imagine that you're sending the vibrations of this sound through the invisible umbilical. Do this three times.

As you make the sound OM, the baby can feel the same comfort and security that she felt while in the womb.

Grounding

Giving birth can be an intensely physical and emotional experience, to say the least—as can taking care of your baby all day long. Whether you have a newborn or an older baby, here's a great way to balance your energy and to feel more grounded and clear any time.

- Stand with your feet together, hands at your sides.

- Now cross one ankle over the other, so both feet are on the ground. Whether you choose left over right or right over left doesn't matter; just do what feels best to you. (fig. 1)

- Now, with your arms straight down, bring your palms together, crossing your wrists the same way you crossed your ankles—left over right or right over left. (fig. 2)

- Fold your arms and hands up so that your hands are even with your chest. (fig. 3)

- Notice the feeling of being grounded and centered in your body.

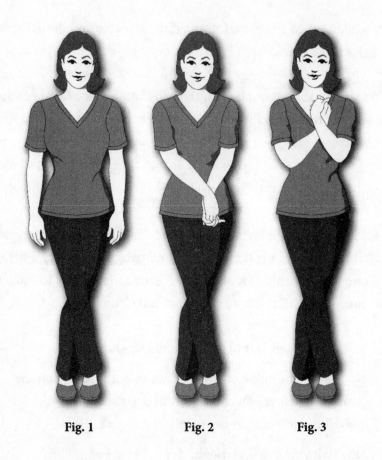

Fig. 1   Fig. 2   Fig. 3

Eyes in the Back of Your Head

You know that saying that mothers have eyes in the back of their head? When it comes to sensory perception, that's very true. Many mothers talk about a "sixth sense" they feel when it comes to their baby—an innate sense of *knowing* about the baby that isn't connected to the five senses of seeing, hearing, touch, taste, or smell.

Connecting to yourself and your baby regularly by working with CALM can help make you more aware of that sixth sense, or intuition, and here is another exercise you can try. Place the baby in front of you, in her carrier or on a blanket on the floor. Now focus on the baby, but expand your field of vision to include your peripheral vision as well while you continue to look at the baby in front of you. Now see if you can stretch your awareness to sense things in the room beyond what you can actually see. Take this one step further by expanding your field of reference to fill the entire room, including what is above you, below you, and behind you. Can you *sense* the furniture and objects throughout the room, even though you can't see them? As a mom, this heightened level of perception can serve you very well!

Attunement

Some degree of misattunement is actually healthy for a child. If you were to perfectly attune to your baby at all times, she would not only likely feel "crowded" by your hovering but would grow up expecting everyone else to read her perfectly at all times, too, which isn't realistic. D. W. Winnicott, a pediatrician and pioneer in studying mother-baby attachment, defined the "good enough" mother as one who doesn't flawlessly attune to her child at all times but who can stay present with her child through both her positive and negative experiences.[13] Because some misattunement is unavoidable between a mom and a baby, and between the baby and the rest of the world, the self-attunement you model for her is invaluable.

Heart of Gold

This one is a no-brainer—literally. It's all about nudging you out of your head and into your body. Though the steps seem quite simple, this meditation can bring a profound sense of peace and joy. Research shows that meditation and visualization can help you relax, lower stress, and improve focus, even when multitasking.[14] The calm that can result also signals to the brain that you are safe and all is well.

- Imagine that there is a seed of gold light at the center of your heart.

- Take a deep breath in, imagining that the gold light slowly expands to the size of a chestnut, then an apple, then fills your heart, and then travels slowly throughout your entire body.

- Continue to breathe deeply, seeing your body completely filled with gold light.

- *Optional*: Visualize the gold light expanding from your heart center to just outside of your body until it reaches and envelops your child, whether she's physically present with you or not. If you wish, you can allow the light to fill the entire room, then your home, your neighborhood, and beyond. Intend that the gold light brings a sense of peace, calm, and balance to all that it touches.

To listen to a recorded version of this meditation, please visit our website at www.calmandhappy.com.

Additional Tools for Calming

Every mom sometimes feels stress or frustration in the course of her busy day. If you find yourself losing your cool, take a brief "time out" by choosing one of the options below.

One Minute or Less:

- Take one to three big, giant, deep breaths.

- Scan your body for tension and bring your focus to those areas. Take a few deep breaths as you do.

- Put on some high-energy music and dance like a fool around the living room. The resulting endorphins will lift your mood and help you feel calmer afterward, and you'll probably give your baby quite a good laugh!

- Get some fresh air. Roll down or open the window and breathe deeply.

- Take a quick walk around your yard or garden. Nature has an amazing way of calming and grounding us.

- Just start smiling. Sounds hokey, but by using your "smile muscles" you will trick your brain into thinking that you are already in a lighter mood.

Five Minutes or Less:

- Call a good friend and tell her you only have a few minutes to talk, but you just need to vent. Don't call someone who will judge you in any way but rather a friend who "gets it" about being a mom.

- Alternatively, send an "I'm having one of those moments" e-mail.

- Go to the bedroom or bathroom and close the door—making sure your child is safe, of course (such as in her crib or a playpen)—and just sit quietly, or thumb through a magazine.

- Focus on the sensory sensations you're experiencing in your environment, wherever you are—the sounds you hear (the children's laughter as they play on the swings at the park), the details of what you see (sand and brownish grass, a giant tree with big green leaves), the way the air or sun feels on your skin. You'll be so busy focusing on these other things that your mind won't have room to loop stressful thoughts.

- Watch a funny video online—or maybe a quick snippet of a TV show that always makes you laugh.

- Recall the last time you felt close to your child, and replay that movie in your internal theater. Remember the warm, delicious feelings you had as you were connecting. Your brain doesn't know the difference between what's real and what's imagined; as far as it's concerned, if you're playing the movie it's happening *now*.

Thirty Minutes or Less:

- Take a relaxing bath or a hot shower. If you don't have a candle handy, at least dim the lights. Put on some adult music—you know, the stuff you *used* to listen to before you became a mom.

- Get your body moving: go for a walk or a run, or do a few yoga stretches or poses on your living room floor.

- Take a "mini-vacation." While the baby is napping, grab a juicy novel and an icy cold or hot drink, and curl up in a comfortable, cozy spot. *Do not* answer the phone or check your e-mail for the entire thirty minutes!

- Download and listen to one of the free meditations on our website (www.calmandhappy.com).

- Ask your partner or spouse, or a friend or caregiver, to watch the baby. Go to a nearby café, order your favorite drink, and simply sit and watch the world go by. Resist the temptation to keep texting whoever is watching the baby!

- Catch up by phone or video chat with a good friend or close relative you haven't connected with for a while. Do this while the baby is napping, or when someone is watching her.

Reflecting Experiences

When your child does something awkward with her body—getting an arm stuck while trying to roll, face planting while learning to crawl, taking a spill as she's learning how to stand on two legs—she's asking you a question: *How should I react, mom?* If you immediately react with concern and panic—"Oh no! Come to mommy and let me hold you!"—chances are good that she will begin to cry and become upset, because that's what you seem to be expecting her to do. If you go to the other end of the spectrum, insisting "You're okay!" you'll have completely glossed over her feelings about what happened. If you simply reflect the experience back to her, though, either through your eye contact *(I saw that)* or by narrating what happened ("Your legs got tired because you're working so hard on walking!"), you'll often find that your child simply dusts herself off and continues on. Try to stay loving but neutral until you can gauge her decision about how *she'll* choose to react. If she's genuinely hurt herself or does become upset, offer plenty of comfort and mama love.

CHAPTER 4

In Search of
Mother Instinct

How Self-Doubt and Negative Thinking Cause Stress

The Road to Disempowerment

Given all of the moving parts that parenting involves—babies are constantly growing and developing, so their needs, moods, and behavior are constantly changing—it's no wonder that moms tend to worry about all the decisions there are to be made. What kind of bottle causes the least gas, and is greenest? Are you putting your child at risk by vaccinating her, or is there a greater risk by *not* vaccinating? When your baby won't sleep, do you let her "cry it out," or pat and shush while she's trying to learn? Every expert who weighs in on any given parenting subject tells you something different, and your mother, mother-in-law, pediatrician, and mommy friends all give conflicting advice, too. It's enough to make your head spin!

We are living in an age when moms have more access to information than ever before. There is the Internet; there are countless books offering parenting advice; there are parenting groups and Mommy and Me classes, where parents can discuss everything from poop to sleep. This relatively newfound availability of information has been beneficial in some ways; for one thing, it allows moms to get quick answers to a wide variety of questions—for example, how to start feeding solid foods or how to increase a baby's tolerance for tummy time. But all of that information can also seem overwhelming, because it's often contradictory. One website says to start solids at four months, while another says to wait until six months. One developmental expert says that you should expose your child to a wide variety of multisensory toys, while another says not to overwhelm your baby with too much stimulation. Who's right, and who should you believe?

The answer seems obvious when you think about it: Lots of the information out there has some merit, but it has to be adapted and applied to each individual baby, mom, and family according to their needs and preferences. For example, a five-month-old baby who's tracking mom and dad's every bite of food might gobble down solids on the first foray, whereas another baby the same age who isn't quite ready may

> Lots of the information out there has some merit, but it has to be adapted and applied to each individual baby, mom, and family according to their needs and preferences.

cough and gag and spit them out. One six-month-old baby might be able to tolerate a few minutes of frustration before settling herself into sleep, whereas another might have a more sensitive nervous system that still causes her to experience frustration as intense distress. In other words, there's no one right answer for all parents and babies all of the time; what's right for your baby wouldn't necessarily be right for another, and vice versa.

Consider this scenario:

Baby Kate is crying. Her mom, Gemma, fed her only an hour ago, so she feels like Kate shouldn't be ready again so soon. And yet Gemma has a funny feeling that Kate is somehow still hungry. But since this doesn't make logical sense, and since her mother-in-law told her that she was overfeeding the baby, Gemma dismisses the feeling. Instead, she picks up the baby and tries to burp her again, even though she got several good burps after the baby fed earlier. She changes her diaper, but the diaper isn't wet. Baby Kate's crying and Gemma's anxiety are escalating by the moment; Gemma bounces the baby on the bouncy ball, puts her in the swing, and even takes her for a walk outside—but still Kate continues to fuss. Finally, Gemma offers the breast again, and Kate not only calms immediately but seems to be sucking vigorously. After a good feeding, she falls asleep.

Later that evening, when Gemma pumps, she notices that she's produced less milk than normal. When she thinks about it, she realizes that she's been much more on the go with the baby the last couple of days; therefore, she hasn't been all that relaxed during feedings and hasn't pumped as often as she usually does. It seems her milk supply has taken a bit of a dip, which means Kate might not be getting as much as she's used to. There are steps Gemma knows to take to attend to this—she'll feed and pump more often for the next few days, maybe even taking some fenugreek or lactation-promoting tea for an extra boost. What she realizes, though, is that Kate was in fact hungry when she was so fussy earlier in the day. Gemma's instinct was right, but she ignored it.

For many moms, sometimes all throughout any busy twenty-four-hour period, their instinct rises up and then gets dismissed. When this happens, mom has effectively disconnected herself from her own guidance; she has chosen to reject her inner sense of what might be best, possibly in favor of another, external source instead. What possible outcome could there be to this choice *other* than stress, anxiety, and worry?

The problem is not that there's too much information available; it's that parents aren't always exercising discernment about whether that information is right for them and *their* baby. Instead, so-called experts—doctors, therapists, child development specialists, and the like—are put on pedestals, as if they have all the answers. (Admittedly, our own clients have put us on this pedestal at times, too, though we always remind them why that's not a good idea.) Sometimes when a mom follows an expert's advice, things turn out incredibly well—hooray! But have you ever had the experience of following an expert or professional's advice to the absolute letter, only to find that the baby still doesn't sleep, still seems gassy, or still doesn't stop crying even though you followed all of the instructions? What we've noticed is that this is far more likely if a parent has become so invested in the

> The problem is not that there's too much information available; it's that parents aren't always exercising discernment about whether that information is right for them and *their* baby.

other person's opinion that they've forgotten to add their own innate feeling of what's best into the mix.

It's not that the outside information isn't valuable; it's that it's valuable only to the extent that it feels right to *you*. When you put too much stock in another person's guidance and not enough in your own, you might as well physically hand your baby over to that person and say, "You know best; you take care of her, because I just don't know how." In your tougher moments, that might even feel tempting! But when you disempower yourself this way, the baby looks around to find you and can't. She then says, "Hey, Mom—where'd you go? And why am I sitting at the feet of this strange person I don't know, who says I'm supposed to be crawling by now even though I'm not ready yet? Doesn't she know I'm working on language right now?"

Instinct Versus Fear

In this book we've talked a bit about a mom's sixth sense about the safety and well-being of her baby; that instinct is necessary to ensure a baby's survival. Whether you call it sixth sense, instinct, or intuition, what we're really talking about is a mom's inner sense of what's best for her child. But as we've talked about previously, because of the sympathetic nervous system's fight-flight-freeze response to perceived physical or emotional danger, that intuition is very difficult to access when you are feeling stress and fear but much more accessible when you're relaxed and in the flow of connection and rapport with yourself and your baby. The idea is not that a mom should *never* have fear or pay attention to it; there may indeed be times when you feel genuinely concerned for your baby and immediately take action to protect her, for example by seeking medical attention if a fever spikes.

What's challenging for many moms, though, is differentiating between what's truly your mama instinct and what's actually just the projection of worry about the baby based on your own fears. Because your past comes alive in the present as a mom via those old home movies, *you* may well be in crisis because painful emotions—anxiety, sadness, anger—are coming up in the here and now, but the baby may actually be just fine. How to tell the difference?

Believe it or not, there is very little difference between the energy behind a valuable piece of information that arrives in a moment when you need it (*I think the baby might be crying because she needs to burp*) and an emotional surge that sends you into panic (*She's crying, and I have no idea what's wrong!*). In fact, the *only* difference between the two is that the first results from being relaxed and centered in your body (and connected to your mama instincts), and the second results from being in fear and in your head (and disconnected from your mama instincts). It's really that simple. In the scenario with baby Kate, the information about why she was crying was actually available to Gemma almost immediately; she just glossed over it because she was afraid that her mother-in-law might be right that she was overfeeding the baby. Had she been able to stay more relaxed as the baby started to fuss and then tuned in to see how she could best help Kate in that moment, she likely would have gotten all kinds of interesting and accurate information—and saved herself and the baby lots of trouble.

Any voice in your head that criticizes your choices and decisions and tries to erode your authority and wisdom as a mom is not to be trusted.

The disconnection and resulting self-doubt that many mothers unfortunately experience, some on a regular basis, carry a high price. The fear that both causes the disconnection and results from it feeds into the idea that what is happening—including what you are doing, saying, feeling, or experiencing—is somehow "wrong"; that you're failing as a mom, that harm is going to come to the baby because you're letting her down, that if you don't attend to her in just the right way she won't feel loved, that if you get it wrong she might not love you. The list goes on and on. But any voice in your head that criticizes your choices and decisions and tries to erode your authority and wisdom as a mom is *not* your own voice; that isn't your mother instinct at all, and it is not to be trusted.

A lot of moms—and unfortunately, a lot of people—have a similar habit of fear-based thinking, too, passed down through the invisible umbilical from *their* parents (who inherited it from their own parents, who inherited it from their own parents, and so on). Those habits then became part of the programming that got downloaded onto your blank hard drive when you were a child and were then reinforced by experience. When you second-guess yourself, you can't enjoy your parenting experience; instead, you feel lost, confused, and anything but calm. Your stressful thoughts cause your muscles to tighten and your breathing to become shallow, and the fight-flight-freeze response sends stress hormones into your system and takes you to a state of high alert. Depending on how worked up you get, you may feel anything from mild worry to overwhelmed—and even outright panic.

What does it feel like for the baby when you judge or blame yourself because she is crying or because you can't get her to sleep or to feed? (And by the way, we're not talking about the normal feelings of uncertainty that most moms experience when in unfamiliar territory as a parent; everybody has those.) Your baby loves you no matter what, of course, but because of the invisible umbilical, what you say to yourself silently you might as well be saying to your baby out loud, because she feels every bit of it *as though you are saying it to her*. When you feel negative emotions and your body has a physiological response, your baby then picks up on that negativity, feeling what you feel. If you really embraced that idea, would you want to make a different choice instead?

It's All Wrong

It is not possible to be trusting of our instincts and fearful, calm and stressed, connected and disconnected at the same time. It's an either-or choice; when we focus on one, the other fades. You might also have noticed that both negativity and positivity feed on themselves. This is why the more worried and anxious you get, the more each tends to amplify, and it's also why when you start to lift up into more positivity, you feel better and better. For most of us, where we put our focus is largely unconscious; we're not really aware of how we let fear-based, limited thinking sneak in, sending us higher up the stress-o-meter. Let's shine a little light on how this happens.

As you know by now, when you are disconnected from yourself—meaning checked out of your body and in your head—you're basically left with your thoughts, and the longer you spend time with your thoughts, the more likely those thoughts will become negative. That's just the way the mind works. Your most frequent negative thoughts will generally contain the same themes as the title of your most frequently played internal movies; these are otherwise known as your core beliefs (*People Don't Support Me; I'm Only Loved if I Please You*). The mind's job is to bring you evidence that supports whatever you believe, whether positive or negative. So if you have a movie you tend to play often—that is, a belief—called *I Always Do It Wrong,* for example, your mind will get busy producing thoughts that match it: *The baby*

didn't nap well again—it must be because I put
her down too early or too late, or because I
should have fed her beforehand, or because I
forgot to darken the room. It's all my fault.
Now, it may be true that the baby didn't
nap well because there's something in her
schedule or environment that needs adjusting, but a mom who generally trusts herself
would simply tune in, make the adjustment, and
see what happens next. A mom who doesn't trust herself, on the other
hand, would judge herself harshly and get stuck in a negative thought-
loop. What's sometimes easy to forget is that just because you think
something doesn't make it true.

The mind's job is to bring you evidence that supports whatever you believe, whether positive or negative.

In our work with moms, we've noticed that there are three overarching thoughts, or negative "mama mantras," that tend to cause lots of
stress. They are:

1. *I'm doing it wrong* (and I'm causing my child to suffer).
   This thought is the encapsulation of all the ways that you
   may judge yourself harshly as a mom.

2. *You're doing it wrong* (and you're causing me and/or my
   child to suffer). "You" could be your husband/partner,
   your caregiver, your mother or mother-in-law, your pediatrician, and even your child, for instance when you get
   frustrated that she's throwing tantrums or waking too
   early in the morning. It could also be the water pipe that
   bursts in your ceiling, or the thunderstorm that wakes the
   baby at 3 AM.

3. *Things went wrong in the past or will go wrong in the future*
   (and thinking about these events is causing me to suffer

now). For a new mom, thoughts about the past usually center around childhood issues with your own mom and dad—things they did as parents that you wish they hadn't, things they didn't do that you wish they had. Thoughts about the future contain all the worry about "what ifs": *What if the baby doesn't gain more weight? What if she's getting a cold?* Another variation on this one is, *I might do something wrong in the future*, a common one for new moms who feel like they are often navigating unfamiliar waters.

Power Struggling with Life

What negative mama mantras have in common is that they aren't just neutral commentary on events; instead, they carry the idea that whatever is happening (or happened in the past) should be *different* from whatever is happening (or happened in the past). When you entertain negative thinking, you are power struggling with life, because you are fighting what is—and trying to control what you can't.

Examples of *I'm doing it wrong:*

- I can't believe I didn't see the baby's tooth coming in. She was in pain, and I didn't help her.
- The baby is crying, and I can't get her to stop. I'll bet everyone in this restaurant hates us.
- I never have quite enough milk for the baby. I feel like I'm letting her down.

- We're running late again. It's terrible that I can't seem to get out the door on time.
- I'm the only mom I know who can't get her baby to nap.

Examples of *You're doing it wrong:*

- My mother-in-law should call or come over more often.
- My husband barely helps with the baby. I have to do everything.
- Why won't the baby nap? She needs her sleep!
- The doctor never listens to my questions.
- I can't believe the car broke down again.

Examples of *Something went wrong in the past/Something will go wrong in the future:*

- *Dad was never there for me.*
- *Mom should have trusted me more.*
- *I wish my family had been closer.*
- *What if we can't afford to save for the baby's college fund?*
- *What if the baby's cough gets worse?*

It may be that thoughts like these contain some truth; for example, your father may not have been around as much as you would have liked when you were growing up. What's more important, though, is how dwelling on that thought makes you feel.

Some moms, we've found, tend to focus on one of these thoughts more than the others; *I'm doing it wrong* is usually the most common. Other moms may entertain some version of all of these thoughts throughout the course of their day, one after the other, in an endless stream. Whether you succumb to negative thinking a little or a lot, though, what you may not realize is the direct correlation it has to feeling stressed. Negative thoughts lead to stress, and stressed-out mamas tend to run a lot of negative thoughts through their minds. Negative thoughts also lead to negative emotions, like anxiety, sadness, and anger, and negative thinking plus negative emotion equals even *more* stress. (By the way, negative emotions aren't bad and don't do harm unless we avoid them or hang onto them, which most of us unfortunately do. We'll talk more about emotions in Chapter 7.) The stress that comes from negative thinking and negative emotion also zaps your energy—*far more* than the physicality of taking care of your child—and can affect your physical well-being (including your weight, your milk supply, and your immune system), your ability to be fully present with and attuned to your baby, your other relationships, and your overall outlook on life.

Consider this scenario:

> *Sara, mom to eight-month-old Theo, is exhausted and frustrated. She's done everything she can think of to help Theo nap, but every time she tries to put him down, he starts to wail. Sara feels resentful that the babies of some of her mom friends nap an hour or two at a stretch, whereas she's lucky to get a half hour. She feels angry at Theo and incredibly guilty for feeling this way.*

Whether you succumb to negative thinking a little or a lot, what you may not realize is the direct correlation it has to feeling stressed.

Although it *looks* like Theo's short naps are the cause of Sara's frustration, it's actually her negative thoughts about the situation that are causing her to feel that way—one or more of the negative mama mantras. Feelings are always preceded by at least one negative thought, even if you aren't aware of it, and even if it flashes by in a nanosecond.

If Sara were to examine her thoughts about Theo's naps, here's what she might find:

- *I should know how to help Theo sleep. Why can't I figure this out?* (negative mama mantra no. 1: *I'm doing it wrong*)

- *I've spent hours rocking and holding Theo, and he just refuses to go down.* (negative mama mantra no. 2: *You're doing it wrong*)

- *If Theo doesn't nap, it's going to affect his brain development.* (negative mama mantra no. 3: *Something will go wrong in the future*)

- *All the other moms I know have babies who nap well. I'm the only one whose baby doesn't.* (negative mama mantra no. 1, *I'm doing it wrong*)

- *I'm a terrible mom. I can't get my baby to nap; it's too hard.* (no. 1, *I'm doing it wrong*)

Do you see the spiral of negative thoughts leading to negative feelings leading to more negative thoughts? Focusing on negativity takes you into victimhood; the idea is that there's something "wrong," and nothing you can do about it. That's absolutely never true, because you can always change your perspective.

Fear-based, negative thoughts distort your picture of reality, often making things seem far worse than they actually are; they're like bratty children, taunting you to get a rise. On the playground, a couple of bullies can all too easily incite others to join in—and the same thing happens with negative thoughts, too. While getting Theo up from yet another short nap, here's how Sara could get out of her head and respond rather than react. She would:

- **Cancel negative thoughts** (i.e., *I'm a terrible mom for not being able to figure out Theo's naps; Why the $#%! won't he nap longer?*) by taking a big, deep breath in and releasing those negative thoughts with her exhale breath.

- **Allow her feelings** by focusing on whatever physical sensations and emotions were present, describing them with as much detail as possible. Here's what she might notice:
  - *I just feel incredibly frustrated. There's a lot of tension in my stomach, and it feels hot, like lava.*
  - *My heart is pounding in my chest. I can feel my pulse throbbing in my throat, shoulders, arms, and hands.*
  - *I have a headache—it's in the middle of my forehead, like a big heavy gray block.*
  - *There's a tingling feeling in my hands. It's a little bit prickly and itchy.*

  Sara would take some big, deep breaths right into the places in her body where she felt more tension or emotion.

- **Link up and listen** as she connected with Theo via the invisible umbilical, with the intention of sharing her love and tuning in, not fixing. Sara would gather information with her five senses and her mama instincts, too, continuing to monitor her own body sensations as well.

- **Mirror.** Sara would then mirror back to Theo whatever she noticed, such as:
  - *Hmm, you definitely still seem tired. There's a big yawn, and your little eyelids are all red.*
  - *You sound pretty darn frustrated. You probably want to nap as much as I want you to, but you just don't know how.*
  - *You're hot and damp. I wonder if you're too warm in your sleep sack?*
  - *I'm really not sure how to help you, sweetie, but I'm doing my best to understand what you need.*

As Sara started to relax a bit, who knows—maybe Theo would, too. But even if he didn't, Sara would have much clearer access to her guidance about what might best help Theo with his naps. Here's what she might realize:

- *I think I'm waiting too long to put Theo down. He usually starts yawning and rubbing his eyes a good twenty minutes before we're starting his routine.*
- *I'm going to ditch the sleep sack.*
- *Whenever I get him up from his nap, he's looking over at the window. I'm going to make the room as dark as I can so the light coming in doesn't keep him awake.*
- *I've been pretty stressed and anxious about Theo's naps. Maybe taking some deep breaths throughout the wind-down routine would help us both relax.*

Or Sara might realize, *I really don't know what Theo needs to be a better napper—I need some help with this one.* She might then decide to call a mom friend for advice or hop online to scout around for information. Lots of ideas; lots more empowerment for Sara.

What You Believe Matters

Because your little bright light is so attuned to you, the beliefs you hold about her are powerful. If you believe that you have a "difficult" baby (one who fusses or needs to be held a lot) or that she'll never sleep, guess what? You may inadvertently be contributing to that behavior. Even if you've had lots of similar experiences with your baby where she's behaved a certain way under certain conditions, try to keep an open mind about the possibility that things could turn around anytime, and stay positive. You might be surprised to find that her behavior changes!

Nurturing Your Mama Instincts

Almost all mothers, even those who wouldn't describe themselves as particularly confident, have had at least some experience of *knowing,* from a deep place inside, what the baby needs. For some, these experiences are unfortunately few and far between; for others, they are more common. A mom will tell you that when it happens, though, it's not about thinking about a problem for hours on end. Rather, it's an innate *sense* of what's right in a given moment, almost as if that guidance has been audibly whispered into her ear. Here's an example:

Leah is nursing her baby, Bailey, but she's fussy; she keeps pulling off the breast, arching her back and crying. After trying several times to get her to stay latched on, Leah realizes that she is hunched over Bailey with her breast above, and the milk may be coming very quickly for the baby. Leah adjusts her breastfeeding pillow, sticks another pillow behind her, and leans back a little more comfortably. She takes a deep breath and relaxes a bit, helping Bailey latch on one more time. This time, Bailey begins happily guzzling away, sucking and swallowing easily and rhythmically. All is well.

Some moms, surprised by these instinctive urges, notice them immediately: *Hey, that was interesting—the baby's been fussy at the breast for days, and suddenly I realized that the milk was probably coming too fast.* When a mom focuses on negative thinking, she disconnects from her body and therefore her instincts; when she's in her body and breathing, she is attuned to herself and therefore able to attune to her child and enjoy unobstructed, back-and-forth communication.

Mother's Intuition

Take a few moments to think about the times when you have felt strongly connected to your mom intuition. Maybe you "accidentally" discovered a new burping technique, or maybe you started getting ready to feed the baby moments before she started to fuss. Start paying attention to the times when you sense just what the baby needs; your instincts will become even stronger as you do.

As you are making decisions about your baby's care and well-being throughout your day, the question you want to be asking yourself is, *Am I coming from a place of calm, trust, acceptance, and connection, or one of stress, fear, resistance, and disconnection? Is what's happening with the baby in this moment genuinely requiring an urgent response, or is that just my knee-jerk reaction?* If you're responding out of anxiety and your baby is not in immediate danger, *stop*. If fear is present and there's no genuine urgency, then you have disconnected from yourself, and everything else that happens next—whatever you might do or say—may only add to both your and the baby's distress.

> When you feel challenged in any given moment as a mom, that is your greatest opportunity to center yourself in your body, dig deep into your mama instincts, and *listen*.

When you feel challenged in any given moment as a mom, that is your greatest opportunity to center yourself in your body, dig deep into your mama instincts, and *listen*. Is there anything more precious than the look on your baby's face when she figures out how to do something brand-new? You know this feeling, too; you've experienced it anytime you've struggled a bit in life, then come out the other side having learned a new skill or a valuable lesson. It takes great courage to ride the sometimes turbulent waves of daily life as a mom, and to accept that you may not always know what to do. In Chapters 5, 6, and 7, we'll take a look at the three negative mama mantras in more detail and how using the supports we outlined in Chapter 3, including CALM, can help you find your way.

Surrendering to Uncertainty

Most of us are not comfortable with uncertainty, or "not knowing." Ironically, though, it's surrendering to the idea that you don't know—how to be a mom, how to get your baby to sleep, how best to support her when she cries—that allows you to tune in within and tap into your mama instincts. Spend a few moments thinking about what you do when uncertainty makes you feel anxious. Do you reach for food? Call or text a friend? Distract yourself in some other way? Don't judge yourself for whatever you do; just be aware.

CHAPTER 5

Negative
Mama Mantra No. 1:
I'm Doing It Wrong

*How Self-Blame Causes **Stress***

I f you're like most moms, greeting your baby for the first time brought giant tsunami waves of emotion; as you gazed into the eyes of the precious miracle who had just arrived, you may have felt your heart crack open wider than you ever thought possible. Swooning together inside this new bubble of love, you probably believed that nothing could ever permeate it. And then…the other baby bootie dropped. Within moments, minutes, or hours, the reality of being a new parent set in: *Holy $#%!,* you likely thought, *I'm completely and utterly responsible for this baby's well-being. What if I screw it up?* If you subscribed to that belief, you're unfortunately in very good company. Welcome to parenthood, and the merry-go-round of adoration and worry that most parents ride on a daily basis.

Those dual streams of overwhelming love for your baby and fear about getting it wrong as a parent seem to converge strongly in a mother's heart, and the purpose of this chapter is to help you recognize all of the many ways that being hard on yourself as a mom is causing you stress. In all of our work with parents over the last several decades, we've unfortunately heard lots of different versions of the "I'm doing it wrong" mantra. Even if you feel like you've got a decent amount of confidence and trust in yourself as a mom, in this chapter you're likely going to discover a couple of places in your mind where negative self-talk is hiding.

Remember this scenario from Chapter 2?

> *Since the beginning, breastfeeding has been challenging for Melinda and her baby, Henry. Melinda had always imagined that feeding would come naturally and easily, but Henry has had trouble latching on. Melinda has done her best to help Henry feed better—trying different positions and latch techniques, using nipple shields—and though Henry still struggles a bit, he's starting to gain more weight. But Melinda still feels lots of anxiety when Henry is feeding, and she beats herself up, feeling like she is letting him down. Unfortunately, feeding Henry makes Melinda feel over-the-top stressed, and she and the baby often both end up in tears.*

Over the years we've met many moms like Melinda, who are doing the best they can to attend to their baby but are nonetheless beating themselves up for feeling like they are letting their baby down. Here's how Melinda could work with CALM as she was feeding Henry:

- **Cancel negative thoughts.** Melinda would take a deep breath in, releasing the idea that she is somehow "doing it wrong" by letting Henry down—and any other negative thoughts— with her exhale breath.

- **Allow her feelings.** Because her brain is registering fear and thus triggering fight-flight-freeze, Melinda might be tempted to shut down or check out emotionally. Instead, she would check in and see what emotions were present in her body, as well as any physical sensations—just noticing them, not judging. Here's what she might discover:

  - *There's a whole lot of tension in my arms as I'm holding the baby.*

  - *My back and shoulders feels stiff and uncomfortable.*

  - *This suede couch me makes me sweat so much I feel like I'm in the Amazon.*

  - *There's a big blob of anxiety in my stomach. It's squishy and black and cold.*

  - *There's a kind of pressure in my throat. I think that's sadness. It feels like I might cry any minute.*

  Melinda would take another big, deep breath right into those areas where she felt the most tension and emotion—in this case, her stomach and her throat. If tears wanted to come, she would just let them.

- **Link up and listen.** Now turning her focus to Henry, Melinda would tune in via the invisible umbilical to share her love, and to see what information she could get about *his* experience. Here's what she might discover:

- *Henry's body moves a lot while he's feeding, especially the arm that's free. He likes to kick a lot, too.*

- *His eyes open and close peacefully for a few minutes, but then they squint up when he gets frustrated. Then he pops off and fusses, and his face gets really red.*

- *When he starts to fuss, I feel even more anxiety in my stomach. Wow, lots more anxiety. My heart beats really fast, and it's hard to catch a breath.*

- **Mirror.** Having gathered lots of useful information, Melinda would now reflect back to the baby what she noticed:

  - *"You're working so hard, honey. You can stay latched on for a few minutes, and then you need to take a break."*

  - *"I'll bet you're feeling really frustrated right now. You're hungry and you really want the milk. It just isn't coming as fast as you wish it would."*

  - *"Maybe you're feeling stressed out, too. Let's take some nice, deep breaths together."*

Having connected to herself and the baby and relaxed a bit, Melinda might find that Henry fed a bit more peacefully. Or, an idea or two might pop up: to use a fan while she's feeding or move to a chair that's more comfortable, or maybe to try a variation on a feeding position she'd tried before. If Henry continued to fuss while nursing, Melinda could cycle back through the steps as many times as she needed to, continuing to center herself in whatever she was experiencing. The point isn't to come up with a magical "solution" to every situation you encounter as a mom but rather to stay connected to yourself and the baby, even when the going gets rough.

Remember, negative thoughts lead to negative emotions, which lead to stress. But don't beat yourself up even *more* for having negative thoughts! *All* moms have negative self-talk to some degree or another; for that matter, all human beings do. Just be aware when you are taking yourself down a negative track so you can make a different choice instead.

The point isn't to come up with a magical "solution" to every situation you encounter as a mom but rather to stay connected to yourself and the baby, even when the going gets rough.

The rest of this chapter is devoted to the most common variations we hear on the negative mama mantra *I'm doing it wrong*. See which ones sound familiar!

If My Baby Is Unhappy or Struggling, I Need to Fix It (and if I Can't, I'm Doing It Wrong)

No mother wants her baby to feel pain. When she cries or gets frustrated, you may feel anything from mild concern to full-blown panic, depending on your individual makeup and what's playing in your internal theater. Babies are tiny and largely helpless; they need your assistance for almost everything, and on a primal level, getting their needs met, and you meeting those needs, is about survival. But after about four months, you begin to realize that not every cry is a 911 emergency, and then the lines start to get a little blurrier. When the baby gets frustrated as she's trying to roll or crawl, should you help or stand back and allow a bit of frustration? When she cries, should you continue to pick her up immediately or wait a moment and see if she settles on her own? When she wants to be held as you've got your hands full cooking dinner, should you stop what you're doing and pick her up or tell her she has to wait a minute? Knowing when to assist and when to let her find her own way can be challenging, and many moms end up feeling guilty, frustrated, or anxious if they feel like they can't find the right balance.

You may know very well that attending to the baby in just the right way all the time is mission impossible (not to mention no fun), but the urge to try anyway can be doggedly persistent, despite your best attempts to accept that doing your best to meet her needs is good enough. If you had even a slight tendency toward perfectionism before giving birth, there's a good chance that you watched those seedlings bloom into a full garden of control issues once the baby arrived, because you care so much about her well-being. But even if you felt comfortable tolerating some of the unpredictability and messiness of life before having a child, you may have found that once you became a mother, much to your surprise, you started to sweat the small stuff. That's because once you buy into the belief that you're possibly letting your baby down as a mom ("getting it wrong"), you are bound to want to do anything you can to make things right.

Maybe you're obsessive about your house being clean so the baby won't be susceptible to germs; maybe you track every nuance of her sleep, feeding, and poops, gathering enough data for hours of analysis; maybe you scour one parenting book after another, and the Internet, in

> Even if you felt comfortable tolerating some of the unpredictability and messiness of life before having a child, you may have found that once you became a mother, much to your surprise, you started to sweat the small stuff.

an attempt to discover the magic pieces of information that will ensure that you never fail your child. What you've likely discovered, though, is that the slight feeling of satisfaction you get when you cross these items off of your to-do list is temporary at best—and the anxiety and self-doubt remain, to one degree or another.

What's a worried, loving mom to do?

The Blueprint of Life

All human beings operate according to a universal blueprint of life that says we are attracted to pleasure and averted by pain. You began your own life as a baby according to this blueprint, and your baby follows it, too; it's just the way we're wired as human beings. Following the roads toward pleasure and away from pain, we reach for what feels good and push away what feels bad.

Here's how this blueprint comes into play as a mom: Because you love your child so much, her pain and pleasure have now become your own. Your concern for her well-being causes you to chase after her comfort, success, and happiness and to try to avoid her pain, struggle, and frustration. When it comes to her safety and survival, this dynamic serves you both very well, as it keeps you apprised of any adjustments you may need to make to ensure her well-being. But when it comes to everthing else, you're in for a rough ride, because you are sitting in a boat that rides up and down on the choppy waters of your child's own ups and downs. The truth is that your child doesn't want that kind of responsibility at all; it's way too much pressure. Children who know that they are the cause of their parents' happiness or unhappiness end up feeling afraid, confused, and, ironically, *disempowered* by their apparent ability to control mom and dad's emotions. Feeling

responsible for a parent's happiness or unhappiness is a very heavy burden for a child
to carry.

Feeling responsible for a parent's happiness or unhappiness is a very heavy burden for a child to carry.

You almost certainly know this truth
from the inside out. If you are highly
invested in your child's ups and downs as
a mom, chances are excellent that your parents, consciously or not, were highly invested
in what *you* did as a child, because they were
worried about your pain or happiness and their own. Although there
was undoubtedly plenty of love behind their choices, when parents
want to control their child's life experience, that's actually about fear.
Inevitably, some of your parents' fear, and its resulting patterns of
behavior, passed through the invisible umbilical to you and became
the programming on your hard drive. Let's paint a couple of different
pictures to illustrate this a bit more.

Let's say that as a child you were taught that it was your job to
meet one or both of your parents' needs in just the right way. That
belief, still going strong inside of you now, is spilling over into your
relationship with your own child; today, you believe it's your job to
meet your *child's* needs in just the right way. The problem is, what that
"right way" is isn't usually very clear, because you've found that the
things you do to meet her needs work only some of the time, or maybe
even most of the time—but not all of the time. And since you've set
yourself up for an impossible task—you can't make her happy, or
meet her needs perfectly, all of the time (just as you couldn't with your
parents)—your anxiety likely carries with it a lot of self-judgment and
self-criticism, and that good ol' feeling that you're "doing it wrong."
On a never-ending search for clues about how to "do it right" instead,
you may often look for answers outside of yourself.

In another scenario, as a child you had parents who worried a lot that you might fail or fall. That anxiety led them to hover close by, monitoring your choices and decisions and attempting to manage your life experience. Because you were seldom allowed to struggle, when your own child struggles today you want to control the situation and rescue her out of her frustration, believing that that's the loving thing to do. While love is always part of the equation for a mom, though, it's actually your anxiety that's the primary motivator here.

If either scenario sounds familiar, see if any of these statements also ring true:

- *When my child struggles or is unhappy, it's my job to make it better for her.*

- *When my child struggles or is unhappy, it's my fault—I must have let her down in some way.*

- *I worry about my child a lot—that she doesn't sleep enough, doesn't eat enough, or might be getting sick. If she's not doing well in some way, I feel like a bad mom.*

- *When I'm away from my child, I feel guilty because she might need me and I wouldn't be there for her.*

- *A good mom takes care of all of her family's needs, whatever they are.*

- *I have a nagging sense that I'm failing my child.*

- *I feel like I don't understand how to meet my child's needs.*

- *I rely heavily on the Internet, my parenting books, the classes I take, and other people's opinions to know how to be a good mom.*

- *I worry that my child _____ (fill in the blank).*

- *When someone criticizes my parenting choices, I feel bad about myself.*

- *I often feel anxious, worried, isolated, lonely, empty, or overwhelmed as a mom.*

All of these statements contain the same basic underlying sentiment: *I'm completely responsible for my child's happiness and well-being, and if I fail, I'm letting her down* (i.e., "doing it wrong"). We can just hear your thoughts as you read these words: *Well* of course *I'm responsible for my child's well-being—I'm her mother!* On a primal level, we wouldn't argue with you; it's absolutely true that your child is dependent on you for survival—as well as love, nurturing, and security. But beyond providing for these basic needs, much as you might *wish* you could carve out a perfectly smooth path for her in life—and ensure her success and happiness every step of the way—you can't. And thank goodness, because life would be pretty dull without its twists and turns and ups and downs. Challenging as they may be at times, how would we learn and grow without them and the inevitable struggle and frustration they bring? That struggle and frustration are what motivate us to find creative solutions to life's problems and, consequently, build our confidence and self-esteem. One of our colleagues, Betsy Brown Braun, has a wonderful saying: "Prepare the child for the path, not the path for the child." Much as these words ring true in the hearts of many moms, though, actually living by them is not always easy.

Prepare the child for the path, not the path for the child.

If your mama mantra is some version of *My child is crying/not sleeping/throwing tantrums/not listening/letting others take his toys/*

hitting or biting other kids—and I want to fix it, or *When my child is unhappy, I feel guilty/my heart breaks/it's not fair/I hate to see her struggle—and I want to fix it,* the bottom-line translation is, *What my child is doing or feeling is making me anxious, and it's my own anxiety that I really want to push away, or "fix." But since I can't, I'll try to change my child's feelings, behavior, or experience instead.* Makes sense, doesn't it? And let's be honest: a baby who fusses a lot or sleeps little, or a child going through a challenging developmental stage—particularly one that involves acting out or aggression—is no picnic. But there's a difference between taking steps to help your child navigate through a difficult moment or phase and feeling a sense of urgency to fix things and change the behavior. When you feel a sense of urgency and anxiety about your child's behavior or feelings, that's a surefire sign that you have an emotional investment in what she does or doesn't do—and that's about you, not her.

Are You Controlling Your Child?

Grab a piece of paper and jot down the ways that you tend to reach for control of your child's life experience or react to feeling controlled by her behavior. Seeing these things on paper will help you recognize when these tendencies are coming up for you. Make a note also of how you believe these tendencies are affecting your parenting experience—positive or negative. Take a moment to think about how taking a step back and relaxing control might produce a different outcome.

Attempts to control your child's life experience, far from helping her to succeed, will cause her to have poor self-esteem. Children who are never allowed to struggle, and thus find their way either through acceptance of that struggle or problem solving, never develop the confidence that comes from believing the answers are within their own reach. Have you ever noticed that the people we tend to think of as the most successful—business leaders, talented entertainers, and star athletes—also tend to have life stories peppered with all kinds of struggle? The multimillionaire was once destitute; the award-winning actor had a childhood riddled with pain and tragedy; the philanthropist who works tirelessly to support people with cancer is a cancer survivor herself. It is one of life's ironies that the thorniness and anguish of pain can sharpen a person's focus and resolve to rise above it, building character and feelings of self-worth.

Signs That You May Have Control Issues with Your Child

- You get irritable or angry when your baby doesn't comply with your wishes.

- You keep replaying in your head an interaction with your child after the fact, focusing particularly on what you did or said, or didn't say or do.

- You want to mediate if your baby takes a toy from another baby or allows her toy to be taken—even if neither baby is upset.

- You feel irritable or anxious when your baby does something unexpected that affects your planning, such as taking a short nap or getting sick.

- You have difficulty tolerating "messiness"—clutter in the house, lots of big feelings (in you or your baby), deviations from your normal routine.

- You get into lots of power struggles with your older baby who's testing limits.

- You worry about everything—whether your baby might be getting sick, whether she ate enough for lunch, whether she's cold at the park without her jacket, whether she's as social as other babies.

Letting Go of Control

No one else has the power to give you happiness or take it away, and you don't have that power over others, either—including your baby. Instead, each of us is responsible for our *own* happiness—including your baby. This doesn't mean that you won't offer help when she's struggling; it just means that you're checking to make sure it's not your anxiety that's motivating you, and that you're not giving yourself a report card based on her mood: an A+ if she's happy, an F if she isn't. What you can also commit to is staying connected with her regardless of what is happening; the message "I'm right here with you while you're having this experience," from the mirroring step in CALM, is a powerful and loving offering.

The Road to High Anxiety

Here's a sneaky way that your mind may get you to buy into "I'm doing it wrong": *Oh no. I just had a negative thought. Did my baby hear it? Did she feel it? Have I harmed or damaged her in some way? Is she going to start thinking negatively because I did? What if she's hearing and feeling these thoughts, too, right now?*

If you'd like to travel the road of high anxiety and lots of stress, feel free to entertain thoughts like these. Or, you could choose a much more peaceful track instead: *Oh look, there's that negative thought again—the one that always pops up and says I'm doing it wrong. Boy, am I tired of having that thought. Who says I'm doing it wrong, anyway? I'm doing the best I can, and doing my best is what being a loving mom is. Since my baby and I are so connected, the less I beat myself up and the more I honor and respect myself, the better I'm modeling for her how to believe in herself, too.* Which path sounds better?

I Don't Know What's Best for My Child (and if I Don't Seek Advice from Someone Else, I'm Afraid I'll Do It Wrong)

Every new mom is constantly finding herself in a situation she's never been in before. Even if you're not a first-time mom, you've never parented *this* child before, and you may be surprised to find that this baby's needs are very different from those of your other child or children. All of that uncertainty can cause a mom to feel confused at best, if not pretty darn anxious.

That confusion, uncertainty, and anxiety is what causes many moms to get into the habit of looking "out there"—to others—for answers about what's best for their child, sometimes before searching inside themselves first. And let's not forget all of those people—perhaps other moms, your family members, the "parenting experts," or your pediatrician, for instance—who are wagging their finger at you, insisting that they know what's best for your child. But consider this: the degree to which you give credence to those outside voices *over your own* is a direct reflection of your self-esteem.

> The degree to which you give credence to those outside voices over your own is a direct reflection of your self-esteem.

The stronger your sense of self, the less susceptible you are to outside influences; the less self-worth you have, the more stock you will put into others' opinions and ideas. That is not to say that a balanced mom won't consider other opinions; it's wise to do so, especially when you're dealing with a particularly thorny parenting issue—for example, your baby is biting other children on playdates. But there's a difference between taking in outside information—whether from friends, professionals, books, or the Internet—and worrying that you don't know the right thing to do as a parent but someone else does. The more you entertain the latter idea, the more likely you are to find yourself running in circles or changing your mind every time a new, better-sounding opinion comes along. That chase can be dizzying.

Because so many moms either don't live near their extended families or experience some level of disconnect in those relationships, this other cast of characters, for better and worse, seems to have cropped up in their place. There are some wonderful things about this development—for instance, a parenting-group leader may be able to flag a mom's postpartum depression—but in general there's way too much focus on others telling mom how she should be going about her parenting and way too little in the way of supporting her to find her own way. Think back for a moment to a time when you really wavered about a decision; maybe you weren't sure if you were ready to take an overnight trip with the baby, or maybe you were considering moving her from sleeping in your room to her own. Did you waffle back and forth between your options, circling in loops as you worried about what would be best? If so, how did that feel? Pretty stressful, most likely. Now think back for a moment to those times when you simply *decided* to take action as a mom, even if you weren't sure of the outcome. How did *that* feel? What we've noticed is that when a mom grounds herself in the confidence of a decision she makes, even when she doesn't know how it will turn out, the baby feels safe and well cared for and will often fall right in line with whatever mom decides. Maybe the baby even helps to co-create those choices you make when you're more relaxed, communicating with you through the invisible umbilical.

> When a mom grounds herself in the confidence of a decision she makes, even when she doesn't know how it will turn out, the baby feels safe and well cared for.

Getting still enough to hear your own voice is, of course, the challenge—especially when you hit the ground running on a daily basis and there's barely a moment to breathe, let alone be still. That's why the aim of this book is to help you do just that—not as one more thing to add to your laundry list but as an important foundation to your best functioning as a mom.

"My Child Knows Best"

This is absolutely true—for the first four months of life. Pediatrician Harvey Karp, author of *The Happiest Baby on the Block,* dubbed the first four months the "fourth trimester" because human babies are born far less developed than babies of other species; they need quite a bit of care and assistance early in life.[15] In that first four months, it is vitally important to follow a baby's lead in terms of feeding, sleep, and overall caretaking; this promotes healthy attachment. Your consistent response also helps a baby learn how to regulate her own internal systems, which she'll be able to do more and more of, slowly, after the cognitive milestone that usually peaks between three and four months.

As your baby grows, she can start to become increasingly more independent in some ways—in incremental steps and stages. At the same time, while it remains important to respond consistently to her needs, you can start to take the lead in certain key areas. For instance, while she may prefer to play patty cake with you when she wakes at 3:00 AM, you are not obliged to accept the invitation to that party! Similarly, if your baby continues to fuss and cry every time you put her down, you can begin to slowly help her increase her tolerance for downtime, even if she's not a huge fan of that idea—and even if it's only a few minutes at a time.

In the bigger picture, as she grows and develops, it's true that your child's best compass for navigating life lies within. But if children always knew what was best, they wouldn't need parents. Beginning to discern between what your child *wants* and what she *needs* is a challenging terrain that every parent must navigate. Like everything else with parenting, there are no hard and fast rules—but as you experiment with finding the balance between following her lead in some areas and taking the lead in others, you'll discover through your experience what works best for you and your baby.

My Doctor Knows Best

Pediatricians have lots of knowledge about your baby's physical well-being: they'll track her weight and height, give plenty of advice for how to keep her healthy, and diagnose and treat any medical issues that may need attention. If you're lucky, your pediatrician may also have some knowledge about things like breastfeeding, eating solids, development, and sleep. Doctors usually aren't taught these subjects in medical school, however, so not all doctors take it upon themselves to become experts in these areas, and one who has a more holistic approach to treating babies isn't necessarily a better doctor. Feeling that there's a good fit with your pediatrician is really a matter of your family's particular priorities and sense of kinship with that person.

We've heard many stories over the years, though, from moms who were told something by their pediatrician that *didn't* resonate with them, and they didn't necessarily feel comfortable speaking up about it—at least not at first. Derek's daughter, Orla, had that experience. When Orla's daughter, Alexa, was eleven months old, she developed a high fever. Orla rushed her to the emergency room, only to be told that the baby simply had the flu and that the best treatment was acetaminophen, lots of fluids, and rest. Orla reluctantly went home, but Alexa's symptoms not only didn't improve, they got worse—and her fever spiked higher.

Back at the hospital, Orla was told that there was nothing more they could do, and she was encouraged to take Alexa back home. Orla now had a dilemma; the medical experts were telling her that her daughter would be okay, but she had a strong feeling that something was definitively *not* okay and that the true source of Alexa's symptoms had not yet been discovered. Unquestionably, part of her skepticism had to do with the fact that this same hospital had told Orla's mother,

Linda, three years earlier that the headaches she was experiencing were due to stress; it was only on Linda's third visit to doctors there that they discovered that she had had a stroke weeks earlier, and because she had not been properly diagnosed and treated, she died due to bleeding in the brain.

Remembering this painful experience and summoning all of her strength, Orla insisted that the doctors had missed something in Alexa's symptoms and refused to leave the hospital until they ran more tests. In the end, doctors discovered that they had failed to diagnose a simple kidney infection. Antibiotics were administered, and Alexa recovered within a few days. Had Orla not spoken up, though, Alexa may well have gotten much sicker than she did.

Although doctors do their best to diagnose and treat children's medical symptoms, they sometimes miss things—and get busy, overwhelmed, and overworked, just like everyone else. In other words, they are human. Fortunately, Orla's experience is not typical, and there is no reason to suspect a doctor is missing something as a matter of course. But if you have a strong feeling about something physically going on with your baby—particularly in a case where symptoms are ongoing—do not assume that the doctor automatically knows best. Ask questions, do your own research, and perhaps consider a second opinion. Above all, follow your instincts if your instincts are telling you that the true cause of your baby's symptoms has not yet been found.

We All See the World
Through a Different Lens

It's sometimes easy to forget that the ideas and opinions of your parents, siblings, extended family, friends, coworkers, spouse, and pediatrician are influenced and colored by their individual experiences. The mom at the park who insists that moms should stay home with their baby may have felt angry when growing up that her own mother worked; the nurse at your pediatrician's office who suggests that good parenting means holding your baby constantly may have had a childhood where she felt neglected by one or both parents. Everyone sees the world through their own lens, and that's why putting more stock into others' points of view than your own is such a slippery slope. If you typed "What should I do when my baby cries?" into your computer, what would happen? Your search engine would bring up all kinds of answers and information, running the spectrum from "pick her up immediately" and "wait a moment and see if she settles" to "let her be so she can self-soothe." Giving more weight to others' opinions about what's best for your baby instead of your own is like asking the Internet for answers to very personal questions about *your* baby.

My Mother/Mother-in-Law/ Aunt/Sister Knows Best

This is a tough one, particularly if Grandma or your other female relative is one of those supermoms who, in your esteem, did a wonderful job as a parent raising you or your husband or partner, or their own kids. When this is the case, it can be extremely tempting to want to simply download all that this mama knows onto your own parenting hard drive and call it a day. And truth be told, if you feel in sync with her advice in most arenas, there is nothing wrong with adapting what she offers into your own parenting repertoire; the key is determining whether you're truly on the same wavelength or whether you're just assuming that she knows what's best for *your* baby because you view her as such a stellar mom to her own. Even if she deserves an award for being Mom of the Century, it's *still* important to weigh what she's offering against your own heart and experience.

Others of you may have a mother or mother-in-law, or other relative, who believes she knows best even if you don't agree. Though you may be aware that you disagree with her, perhaps in certain key areas—such as how much to hold her or how to get her to sleep—it may be tempting, particularly if there is a history of conflict in the relationship, to defer to her just to keep the peace. That's certainly an option, and if you can do so without an emotional charge, then all is well. But if you're quietly seething and keep your mouth shut just to avoid a confrontation, what will happen over time is that you'll build up a bubbling cauldron of resentment that will eventually begin to rise up and threaten to scald everything in sight. For some moms who become grandmothers, the new role brings an awareness of their own aging process, which can cause them—often unconsciously—to assert their authority and, unfortunately, have difficulty deferring to you as the mom and supporting you while you find your way. In other words, offering their knowledge and wisdom gives them a confidence boost at a time when they are feeling vulnerable. Even if you can empathize with the challenges of this life stage, though, this is not your torch to bear.

Whether or not you agree with the advice your mom, mother-in-law, aunt, or sister is sharing, *you* are the mom, and you get to decide whether you follow that advice. "Thank you, I'll definitely consider that!" is a polite but noncommittal response to almost any suggestion, and one that leaves plenty of room for your own exploration of whether what's being offered is right for you.

"The Experts" Know Best

There are many so-called—and self-titled—parenting experts out there, many of whom have written wonderful books, share invaluable tips on social media, have a treasure trove of information on their websites, and teach top-notch classes on their area of expertise. (And yes, some parents have referred to us this way over the years, too.) These professionals, many of whom have years of experience of working with parents and families, include authors, educators, therapists, doctors, parenting group leaders, and media personalities. Without a doubt, lots of these well-intentioned folks have valuable information and experience that can help a mom or a dad gain insight into a particular parenting issue, and in some cases help them resolve long-standing challenges. Unfortunately, though, parents who resonate with a particular expert's language or ideas sometimes tend to put *all* of their eggs into that expert's basket, forgetting that that person is not standing in your shoes (or slippers, depending on the hour), raising your particular child. And besides, no parenting book can tell you how to parent in the moment.

Some of these experts claim to tout *the* philosophy, method, or way of parenting that will infallibly create a happy, healthy, well-adjusted child. If that were actually true, though, then all of the parents following that philosophy or method or way of parenting would have happy, healthy, well-adjusted kids—and as we all know, that isn't quite how it works. There is no *one* magic answer to any one parenting question, nor is there one way of parenting that trumps another; rather, some of the wisdom from the experts can support the foundation upon which you build your own values and priorities as a mom. If you come across information that resonates for you, by all means weigh it, consider it, and try it on—but always bring that information into your own heart to see whether it feels right for you and your baby. You may find that treating the information on the Internet and in books like a buffet—taking what works, leaving the rest—allows you to gather the tidbits that will help make you stronger and more confident without taking on information that could potentially send you down the wrong path for you.

There is no *one* magic answer to any one parenting question.

My Mom Friends Know Best

Yes, they do—for *their* child, not yours. We've heard countless moms over the years report that the mom they met at the park/in the grocery checkout line/at the birthday party/in their Mommy and Me group told them *unequivocally* that a baby should sleep through the night by four months, that if your baby isn't rolling by five months she's developmentally delayed, that feeding your baby nonorganic solids puts her at risk for cancer, and the list goes on. When a mom discovers a tidbit of information, a handy product or gadget, or a schedule that works well for her and her baby, she may become excited and want to share that wisdom with others, usually intending that what's working for her will work for others, too. There's nothing wrong with moms sharing their experience with other moms, of course; the trouble comes when the mom receiving the information takes it as gospel and believes that if what worked for another mom *doesn't* work for her or her baby, she's the one who's wrong. Nope.

Mom-to-mom wisdom is one of the most reliable sources of information out there, because other moms—particularly those with babies roughly the same age as yours or older—are right there in the trenches with you, machete-ing their way through parenthood just like you are. Why reinvent the wheel when someone else has already smoothed and perfected it? By all means, glean as much wisdom as you can from other moms, but just as with every other area, weigh it against what feels right for you and your child. There is no one-size-fits-all answer to *any* parenting challenge or arena.

All the Other Moms Have Motherhood Wired (and Since I Don't, I'm Doing It Wrong)

You've had your eye on her since the very first music class. She's always on time—early, in fact—and you're often late. Her baby smiles constantly and never fusses and is always wearing some cute outfit that miraculously seems immune to spit-up and drool. Your baby, meanwhile, begins to wail the minute the singing gets too loud, and you're grateful if her outfit stays clean for the first ten minutes she's wearing it on any given morning. Just what *is* it about this other mom that makes you both hate her and want to be her at the same time?

If you've ever felt envious of another mom who insists that motherhood is "incredibly easy" or marveled at a mom who fits into her skinny jeans two months after giving birth (no muffin-top pregnancy souvenir in sight), you may be tempted to believe that some of the other moms out there have life with baby all wrapped up with a neat, pink polka-dot bow. But because we have talked to thousands of moms over the last several decades in our work with parents, we have the inside track: Even the mom who *looks* like she's got it all together, and has a baby with an amazingly sunny disposition who sleeps through the night, has her own fair share of stuff going on behind closed doors. She may have a mother-in-law who won't speak to her, or a husband who's been AWOL since the baby's birth; she may be thin, but that's because she's starving herself. In other words, no matter what it looks like on the surface, what you're seeing is only part of the picture, and there is likely plenty going on underneath. *No* mom has it all figured out, and anyone who believes otherwise is comparing herself to someone who doesn't even exist.

No mom has it all figured out, and anyone who believes otherwise is comparing herself to someone who doesn't even exist.

Comparing yourself to other moms usually brings feelings of anxiety, jealousy, shame, and self-doubt. A close cousin of this is comparing your baby to other babies, for example worrying that your nine-month-old isn't standing yet because you know three other babies the same age who are. When comparing yourself with others, you either feel better than they are or worse off. There's no middle ground in this equation; comparison inevitably brings a power differential, and when we disempower ourselves, we then either seek to validate that disempowerment (*It's true; I'm not as good as she is*) or we make the other person smaller to feel our powerfulness again (*I'm actually better than she is*). True empowerment seeks not to separate and compare but to connect and support.

To stay centered and grounded, keep the focus on you and your baby. Avoid the "grass is always greener" mentality of imagining that another mom has motherhood wired; that's like saying that someone has *life* wired, and anyone who has ever held that thought, even for a nanosecond, most likely experienced plenty of evidence to the contrary in the very next nanosecond afterward.

I Should/Shouldn't Think, Feel, or Do _____ (Otherwise, I'm Doing It Wrong)

There are lots of ways to fill in the blank here: I should always want to be with my child; I should always comfort her when she cries; I should be more patient, worry less, feed her organic foods more often. There may be nothing more stressful than the idea that whatever you are thinking, feeling, or experiencing "should" be different from what you are thinking, feeling, or experiencing. While you can address the thoughts and feelings that arise throughout your day, what you can't control is *that* they arise; as you've probably discovered, pushing them away or squelching them tends to make them stronger. When you recognize them as messengers, on the other hand, you can gather information about what's going on inside of you and make any adjustments you wish to make.

It's powerful to simply accept the truth of where you are as a mom in any given moment. Having the thought, *I'm not enjoying being a mom right now* or feeling angry that you didn't get to eat lunch because the baby napped for only twenty minutes doesn't mean you don't love your baby; it just means you're human. Plus, as we've discussed elsewhere, having a baby is like having a living, breathing reminder of your childhood past at all times, meaning that some of your more painful memories— times when you may have felt ignored or rejected, for instance, or struggled while feeling unsupported—may stop you in your tracks. So when your baby gets frustrated because she can't seem to master rolling onto her tummy despite weeks of practice, and *you* feel frustrated that she's frustrated, you are most likely time-traveling into the past and remembering a time when you felt alone in your own frustration. If you're also telling yourself that you shouldn't be feeling that way, you're putting yourself in a no-win situation. You supposedly shouldn't feel something you are in fact feeling, so where can you possibly go from there except into lots of stress?

> It's powerful to simply accept the truth of where you are as a mom in any given moment.

Remember, it isn't that having negative or stressful thoughts at times will harm your baby; it's when you chronically either feed those thoughts with more negativity *or* deny them that you end up influencing your little one's neural programming. What you can do instead is to recognize these thoughts as messengers reminding you that you have options to bring your stress down a few notches. Use one of the support tools from Chapter 3: take a few deep breaths, work with the steps for CALM, or use your anchor. This will help get you out of your head and back into your body—and the present moment.

I Can Do It All on My Own
(and if I Can't, I'm Doing It Wrong)

The notion that a mom should be able to take care of her baby 24/7, be a doting wife, run a perfectly organized household, manage her work schedule if she has one, and give nonexistent leftover time and attention to friends and extended family is a surefire recipe for nonstop stress. Heck, you're lucky if you spin *one* of those plates on any given day. The pressure on moms to be superhuman has been widely discussed in the media over the last two decades or so, but despite all of the hot debate, the myth that a mom can have it all or do it all still persists.

No mom is an island, and yet the idea that a mom needs help in taking care of her child still seems to strike many as a sign of weakness.

When we give too much power to others, we get lost; when we rely too heavily on our own resources, we get stuck. No mom is an island, and yet the idea that a mom needs help in taking care of her child still seems to strike many Western moms as a sign of weakness. "My mom did it all without help, so why shouldn't I?" is a refrain we hear a lot. Even if that's actually true (though often when you scratch the surface, you discover that grandma didn't work, whereas mom does; or that grandma had extended family around her, and mom does not), so what? She isn't you, and if you're feeling isolated and overwhelmed, then that's simply your truth. This section shares threads with every other section that comes before it: a mom who struggles to do it all and can't often tries even harder to control her environment; she may mistakenly believe that all the other moms are "doing it all" and she isn't; she may feel that she doesn't know what's best for her child and isolate socially due to her shame;

and she may insist that she "should" be able to do it all on her own, denying her own struggle in the attempt to appear that she's managing quite well even if she really isn't.

Five Things You Can Do Right Now to Connect:

1. Call or e-mail a friend or family member who will only listen, not judge (choose carefully!).

2. Ask a mom friend to meet you for a stroll, for lunch or for coffee, or for a playdate. If you don't have a lot of mom friends yet, consider taking a class where you can meet other moms, or reach out to another mom at the park.

3. Close your eyes and take a deep breath, imagining that you are connecting with all of the other mothers on the planet; feel their strength, presence, kinship, support, and sisterhood.

4. Look through photos or watch videos of friends and family.

5. Go onto social media or places online where moms are gathering. Shout out.

Moms who are connected to supports in the form of parenting groups, other mom friends, extended family, professionals who can help troubleshoot specific areas of parenting (such as pediatricians and lactation consultants), and who have an open, supportive relationship with their partner or spouse thrive exponentially more than moms who are isolated and struggling. Not every mom who prefers to keep to herself is struggling, mind you; we're referring to the idea that handling every aspect of motherhood on your own is some sort of ideal picture, and whoever paints the picture with the most color wins. In truth, no one wins, including your baby.

It does indeed take a village to raise a child, so it's important to identify your "village people"—whether they live down the block or across the country and are accessible only by phone, video chat, or the Internet—and connect with them on a regular basis. There are three circles of support every mom needs to thrive: (1) The inner circle, which includes *only* yourself and your partner or spouse; (2) the middle circle, which includes your extended family and close friends; and (3) the outer circle, which includes your pediatrician, caregiver, colleagues at work (if working outside of the home), newer mommy friends (including on the Internet), and perhaps your lactation consultant, parenting group instructor, or therapist, if you have any of these. It's important to make sure that you're connected to both people in the inner circle—yourself and your husband—at all times, and ideally you're also connected to *at least* one other person in both the middle and outer circles at any given time as well.

There's no question that it's easier for a mother to relax when she has a solid foundation of outside support, even if she doesn't agree with every bit of advice and wisdom coming her way, because feeling supported helps you stay calm. But even if you are reading this book and unfortunately feeling a distinct *lack* of support from your community, your family, or even any outside source at all, you can't afford to wait for it to come to you. That perspective keeps you dependent on somebody else to do something, and even the most reliable "somebody" out there still can't be counted on all of the time. At the end of the day, *you* are your own very best, most dependable support—or at least you can learn how to be. As a happy side bonus, the more you practice trusting and showing up for yourself, the more likely others are to do the same for you, too.

Who's on Your Team . . . and Who Shouldn't Be?

Because your time and energy are valuable as a mom, it's important to be aware of who in your life is a strong support for you, and who in your life may be draining your energy. To gain some clarity on this, list five people who support you strongly; they don't have to be women—it's fine to include your husband or dad, for instance, if these are close relationships. Whoever makes it onto this list are your go-to people for feeling loved and connected.

1. _____
2. _____
3. _____
4. _____
5. _____

Now name five people who drain your energy. You know who these people are; they're the ones who criticize or second-guess you as a mom or perhaps seem to value their own perspective on your baby's needs more than yours.

After spending time with these individuals, you feel tired, drained, and depleted.

1. _____
2. _____
3. _____
4. _____
5. _____

Knowing your strongest supports and weakest links, you can choose carefully who you spend your time with.

The Real Expert Is *You*

When your mama mantra is any version of *I'm doing it wrong*, you are allowing fear and stress to enter the picture; the more stressed you are—mentally, emotionally, and physically—the less likely it is that you'll be able to access your true mama instincts. What's more, when you criticize yourself you are unfortunately teaching your child that it's okay for her to criticize herself, too; she is always listening to you, whether you're talking out loud or to yourself. Remember, when negative self-talk and stress are present, it's because you have inadvertently *allowed* it in. *You* are the one who decides what movies and messages play inside your head, and how stressed or relaxed you are, no one else: not your

> When you criticize yourself, you are unfortunately teaching your child that it's okay for her to criticize herself, too.

mother or father, not your mother-in-law, not your husband or partner, not your pediatrician or the parenting experts, not your mommy
friends, and definitely not your baby.

When some version of *I'm doing it wrong* pops up, try turning it
around and using one of these positive mama mantras instead:

- *I'm doing my best, with love.*

- *No one else is standing in my shoes; I know what's best for
  my own baby.*

- *Just because [my mother-in-law, my sister, that mom at the
  park] believes that being a good mom is [cosleeping/not
  cosleeping, staying home with the baby/not staying home with
  the baby] doesn't mean it's true for me.*

- *When I don't know something as a mom and take a leap,
  I learn.*

- *Nobody has motherhood perfectly figured out, including me.*

- *I am never alone in my journey as a mom.*

- *Being a loving mom and connecting to my baby are way more
  important than doing it right.*

There is and always has been only one true expert on your child:
you—and your child's other parent, of course. You have the lead role
in this production called "Mom," and you are also the producer, director, and writer of the script. Everyone else—no matter how wise, how
many kids they've had, or how many diplomas line their walls—plays
a supporting role. Your own experience, whether your actions result
in your baby's continued agitation or instant calm, is your very best

teacher, and the challenges you face as a mom are there to help you sharpen your sense of what works best for *your* particular child, both now and as she continues to learn and grow herself. From this perspective, you *can't* get it wrong.

CHAPTER 6

Negative
Mama Mantra No. 2:
You're Doing It Wrong

How Blaming Others
Causes Stress

E verything in life has a flip side, and the natural counter-
point to *I'm doing it wrong* is, of course, *You're doing it wrong*.
Who is the "you" in this statement? Well, that could be just
about anyone—your husband or partner, for instance, when he suggests that taking care of the baby is easier than going to an office, or
when he tries to calm the baby by flying her around the room like an
airplane, after which she spits up most of her last feed. Or it could be

your mother or mother-in-law, who constantly reminds you that "It's okay to let babies cry" whenever she starts to fuss. It could also be your pediatrician, when she dismisses your questions about the baby's weight gain as excessive new-mom worry; the snarky mom in your playdate group, who judges you for using a pacifier; the big barking dog who scares the baby silly; or the guy at the farmer's market stall who wants to offer your baby a crumbly cookie that screams "choking hazard." In a nutshell, "you" are all those people who threaten to impinge on your baby's happiness and well-being—and yours, too.

As a mom, the fear that somehow your baby isn't being properly cared for, or possibly even harmed, is what leads to the idea that another person is doing something "wrong" in your eyes. That fear has its place, of course, and it's rooted in the same place that your mama instinct is, as we talked about in Chapter 4. You're *supposed* to have strong feelings about your baby's well-being, and you're supposed to step in when you are genuinely concerned that she's not okay. The challenge is being able to discern genuine harm from your *idea* that she is being harmed. Example: when dad is tickling her a little too enthusiastically, you feel like jumping in to rescue her with the same level of alarm that you would if a grizzly bear were about to snatch her. That's the amygdala in action.

Remember the three circles of support we talked about in Chapter 5? The closer to your inner circle someone in your life is, the more likely it is that your interactions with him or her will bring up strong feelings, because you care more. And when you add the well-being of your baby into the mix, you add yet another layer of emotional investment. Relationships are like mirrors; they bring up the good in both people and the bad. And when both people are new parents, the volume on both gets turned up even more.

If the thought *You're doing it wrong* is coming up for you a lot, particularly in regard to one person or a couple of people in your life, it's time to take a closer look in the mirror of those relationships to see what—or who—is staring back at you. You might find that out of concern for your child, the protective mama in you has been a bit hard on that person. You might also find that that particular relationship is pushing an old button from the past, which sure doesn't feel fun but may be giving you an opportunity to examine something that needs your attention. The rock-bottom truth is that short of actually hurting your baby, your tendency to label other people's actions "right" or "wrong" usually has more to do with you—and your own history—than it does them. Recognizing this truth can be incredibly liberating, for both you and the other person. It's not that there won't be times when it's important to communicate about something that's not working; it's just that there's a big difference between coming to that conversation with blame and taking responsibility for your *perspective* on what the other person is or isn't doing to your liking.

Your tendency to label other people's actions "right" or "wrong" usually has more to do with you—and your own history—than it does them.

Let's take a closer look.

My Husband or Partner Is Doing It Wrong with the Baby

Imagine this: you talk your husband into letting you sleep in on a Saturday morning, and you happily snooze till the ripe old hour of

7:00 AM. (Once you become a parent, what used to seem early now feels late, pretty much all the way around the clock.) You come out to the kitchen feeling groggy but better rested than you have in weeks, only to recoil in horror as you see him feeding the baby scrambled eggs; you had decided together than you would wait on eggs till after the baby turned one since you're allergic. *How could he?* you think. Without even bothering to greet him good morning—let alone express your gratitude for the extra shut-eye—you jump in and sweep the eggs out of the baby's mouth, scolding him vigorously and thinking to yourself, *If he could let this happen, what else could happen on his watch? I can't trust this guy at all!*

> There's a big difference between blame and taking responsibility for your perspective on what the other person is or isn't doing to your liking.

Maybe you haven't come up against a fumble quite this egregious, but we're willing to bet that there are other things your well-meaning spouse or partner has done since you became parents that have rung your alarm bells, or at the very least have driven you absolutely nuts. You don't hold these grievances against him, of course (ahem), and his stellar characteristics far outshine his flaws, but he is human after all. Here's the thing about relationships: There are always two in that dynamic, meaning two people with different needs, opinions, perspectives, sets of values, and backgrounds—the list goes on and on. It's actually a minor miracle that we ever manage to pair up with someone else at all, as the odds for connecting on more than one level just don't seem that good. And yet it happens all the time: despite all of the pitfalls and risks, people find each other, start a family, and create a life together.

In our work with parents, we've often seen that when a couple has a baby, every crack and flaw is exposed in their relationship. No matter how solid your foundation or how madly in love or well suited to each other you think you are (or at least thought you were before becoming parents), having a baby will test your partnership in ways you could never have imagined. That little habit that used to feel mildly annoying—leaving wet towels in a heap on the bathroom floor, for instance—now feels personally insulting: *All I do is take care of the baby, and he wants me to pick up after him, too?* Your patience dwindles, because you're sleep deprived and overwhelmed by all of the caretaking; you've got a baby to take care of now, and you simply don't have the time, energy, or patience for the needs of another adult.

Here's a sobering piece of information: The things that you and your mate have conflict over are going to continue to come up for the duration of your entire relationship. You are inevitably going to feel frustrated or even downright livid at times; even if your guy is a wonderful dad and partner, he is sometimes going to drive you mad. The question is, what do you do about it? There are three obvious choices:

1. *Let it go*. This can work a lot of the time for things that don't matter much, but it won't work long term for something that keeps coming up and brings a hefty emotional charge with it.

2. *Take it on*. Always an option, though just know that if you're running lots of emotion about whatever is going on, this will probably lead to a mild tiff at best and a knockdown, drag-out argument where you both say hurtful things at worst.

3. *Look in the mirror*. Huh? Well, that's what you're already doing anyway, when the person in front of you is pushing

your buttons. That's what we're suggesting in this chapter, anyway. No matter what else it seems like, when consistent patterns of conflict plus high emotion are coming up in your relationship, the other person is reflecting back something that is going on inside of *you*—most likely, something about yourself or your past that you have ignored/repressed/rejected/squelched/judged/crucified/dismissed. This is the same phenomenon we've been talking about in your interactions with your little bright light.

Here's an example:

Your husband is a loving dad and father, and your heart melts when he makes the baby laugh with his funny faces, tenderly reads her a bedtime story, and lulls her to sleep in his arms. But whenever she cries, he's a bit slow on the draw, to say the least. He takes his sweet time picking her up, and even when he does finally make his way toward her, he moves at what you would consider to be a snail's pace. What's more, even when she screams at the top of her lungs in the middle of the night, he sleeps right through it. One night while opening the mail, you hear the baby fussing in the other room, and you snap. "She's crying!" you shout as you storm in. "Why aren't you picking her up?"

Years ago, there was an episode of *Oprah* where the producers sent a whole slew of moms off to a spa for the weekend, leaving the kids home alone with dad. Whatever mayhem the moms might have imagined would ensue, it was probably worse. One dad didn't change his baby's diaper *for the whole weekend*. Another dad fed his kids pizza for breakfast, lunch, and dinner. When the cameras panned through the homes after the moms had returned, you saw dirty laundry on the floor, piles of dishes in the sink, and general chaos. What you *didn't* see, though, was unhappy kids; on the contrary, they seemed pretty delighted by all the fun they'd had with dad (though in all fairness, part of that may have been because they saw more of dad than usual). The dads, though tired, didn't seem unhappy either; they readily copped to the disarray, gleefully or sheepishly admitting that they hadn't much bothered to try to keep things in order. All in all, no children were broken or harmed, and nobody died.

The point was not that the dads had won some kind of victory; this was only a weekend after all, and if kids and families lived this way all of the time, no one would feel safe, let alone sane—or clean. The point was more to illustrate that, like the title of a popular children's book series, daddies do things *differently*. They're no less competent at parenting than moms are, and certainly don't love their kids any less; they just have their own way of showing that love. Now, we're not saying you can't go ahead and fight the battle about the "right" way to attend to the baby; if you want to try to talk your guy into doing things your way, go right ahead. Just take note of where that choice leads you: toward calm and happiness or toward stress and conflict?

> Letting dad find his won way in his connection with the baby will serve you better than trying to micromanage it.

Does the fact that he doesn't do things the same way you do mean he isn't being a good dad—or just that he has a different perspective on when the baby genuinely needs assistance and what to offer?

As the mom, because you are often so intuitive about what the baby needs, you may perceive your guy as a dad who is too laid back, too nervous, too careless, or too rough. You might also be tempted to believe that his style of parenting is a reflection of some kind of imbalance in his relationship with the baby, or a measure of his love. But here's another perspective: People, and certainly men and women, are simply wired differently, and just as you've (hopefully!) already adjusted to accepting some of these differences in your own relationship with your husband, you can do the same as you observe his relationship with the baby. Letting him find his *own* way in his connection with her—or at least talking about your choices as a couple who is parenting together—will serve all of you better than trying to micromanage or criticizing.

What's important to focus on, though, is what pushes your buttons, because that's about the mirror. If you react to a scenario like the one we described earlier—or any other, for that matter—with a strong emotional charge, there's something in the picture you're seeing that's bringing up your *own* stuff. For example:

- You felt ignored/neglected by one or both parents as a child yourself, and when your husband doesn't respond to the baby the way you'd like him to, it reminds you of your own childhood pain.

- You yourself feel ignored/neglected in the relationship with your husband—perhaps he's been working harder than ever since the baby arrived, for instance—and your perception of how he's responding to the baby (or not) is reminding you of your feelings about how he's responding to you (or not) in the relationship.

- You have a hard time tolerating your baby's discomfort, and it makes you tense when she cries—so when your husband doesn't respond right away, your anxiety hits the ceiling.

Now, it's not very likely that you're going to
be able to sift through all of those possibilities right in the moment of your anger
and get to the bottom of why you're
reacting the way you are. We're also
not saying that your lovely husband or
partner doesn't sometimes make choices
or do things that seem a little odd, mis-
guided, or downright insensitive. But in
any relationship, there's only one person whose
choices or behavior you truly have any say about: *you*. So let's come
back to your choices in a scenario like this one and examine them in
a bit more detail.

In any relationship, there's only one person whose choices or behavior you truly have any say about: *you.*

One choice is to say nothing and quietly seethe. This is a popular
choice among moms for whom getting angry when you were growing
up was either punished or shut down, or where your parents had a
lot of tension or conflict in the relationship that never quite came to
the surface, so you have no reference point yourself for what healthy
conflict, and its resolution, look like.

Another choice is to react with lots of emotion. "Oh my God! The
baby is crying—why aren't you doing anything to help her?" What
is the likely unfolding of events to follow this kind of unleashing?
Your husband may feel bad, swallowing your accusation that he's
"doing it wrong" so that it becomes *I'm doing it wrong* inside of his
own head, or he may get defensive. He may go quiet or fire a missive
back. Your little bright light will hear and witness and experience all
of this, taking it all in—and may reflect what she's sensing by crying
or seeming upset.

Research indicates that babies as young as six months respond to marital discord, even during sleep. Sleeping babies exposed to parents' angry tone of voice showed greater neurological activity in areas of the brain related to stress and emotion regulation. Marital conflict has been shown to affect the quality of parent-child attachment as well.[16]

A third option is to CALM. Yep—this process works with husbands and partners, too! Here's what that might look like:

- **Cancel negative thoughts.** This is a tough one when someone is making you see red. Making this choice doesn't mean you're feeling thrilled about what's happening; rather, it's about avoiding the temptation to buy into the idea that whatever the other person is doing is *wrong*, which is a judgment that leads to disconnect. When emotional pain is triggered, the first temptation is always to disconnect, but that isn't truly what you want, and once you do that, the possibility for a peaceful resolution to the situation begins to drift away.

- **Allow your feelings.** Even if you're upset, resist the urge to explode, shut down, or check out, all of which are fight-flight-freeze responses based in fear. Instead, come into your body, feel your physical and emotional feelings, and *breathe.* You might feel the heat of anger bubbling just underneath the surface of your skin, your heart may feel like it's pounding out of your chest, your palms may feel sweaty, and it may feel like there's so much energy in your body that you could run a marathon. Remember that if you're feeling lots of emotion, that's likely because whatever your husband is doing has caused your inner projectionist to fire up old scenes with similar themes in your internal home theater.

• <u>Link</u> up and listen, *even if this is the last thing you feel like doing.* Watch your tendency to resist this one; your mind will likely want to *fight for being right* (because you're in fight-flight-freeze) rather than seeking to understand his perspective. Instead, stand in his shoes for a moment and see if you can get a read on where he's coming from; if you need more information, ask him why he's making the choices he is. Check out his body language, facial expression, and tone of voice, and try to imagine what he's feeling. As you tune in and listen, you might realize that while you would *prefer* that your husband respond to the baby in a different way, he hasn't actually done anything wrong.

Take Your Own "Time Out"

If something has happened in the interaction with your significant other that's caused you to hit the boiling point, and it seems likely that you might say something hurtful that you'll regret later, take a time out. Go to another room and take some deep breaths, or take a walk before attempting to resolve the conflict. When we're flooded with anger, our amygdala is in charge, meaning that our resources for logical, rational thinking are temporarily, but severely, compromised. If you're at a 6 or above on a 1 to 10 scale, 10 being "I'm so mad I could breathe fire," cool off before continuing the conversation.

- **Mirror.** Now reflect back what you've gleaned about your husband's point of view as you've been connecting and tuning in. Here's what that might sound like:

  - "Miraculously, it just doesn't bother you when she cries. But that doesn't mean you don't care."

  - "I hear you. I'm not really giving you a chance to respond in your own way, because I jump in so fast."

  - "I know you love her and wouldn't let her suffer intentionally."

  If things start to heat up again as you're talking, don't let yourself circle back to digging in to defend your point of view, no matter how tempting that is; instead, keep connection and peaceful communication as the overarching goal. Cycle back through these steps as many times as you need to.

Don't Make It Personal

In his book *The 7 Principles for Making Marriage Work*, John Gottman shares his research findings on one of the most deadly threats to a marriage: attacking the personal character of the other person. For example, rather than simply complaining that your husband didn't take out the garbage, you accuse him of being lazy and selfish to boot— or imply these things. (Kind of like *You're doing it wrong*, with extra sauce on top.) According to Gottman's research, couples who hit below the belt in this way have the highest likelihood of breaking up.[17]

After moving through these steps, you might shake your head and sigh at your husband's choices, but you may be able to put away the big guns. On the other hand, if you still feel upset even after working with CALM, there may indeed be something deeper that you need to address or communicate about. If so, go ahead—but now you'll be doing so from a more grounded and centered place, rather than simply knee-jerk reacting. There's a big difference between having a conversation that leads to one or both of you adjusting something that could use a little adjusting, and making him, or anyone, wrong.

The Opportunity of Crisis

It's easy to see why having a baby can put your relationship with your significant other into crisis, but did you know that crisis is a sign that a relationship is ready to deepen? If you respond to crisis in a relationship by either reacting with lots of emotion or trying to avoid it altogether, you will effectively disconnect from yourself and the other person—and potentially lose the opportunity to take that relationship to the next level. On the other hand, if you welcome the opportunity that crisis brings by facing it head on, even if doing so is painful and difficult, the rewards can be significant; as you continue to communicate about whatever is causing the conflict and work toward resolution, you'll likely feel closer than ever and more freedom to be yourself in the context of that relationship. Your relationship changes dramatically when you become new parents, so give yourselves time to find your footing together.

My Husband or Partner Is Doing It Wrong in the Relationship

The other big area where it's tempting to hold onto *You're doing it wrong* with your husband or partner, of course, relates to your own needs in the relationship. Whether your significant other has perfectly attuned to your needs as a mom since you've both become parents, whether he's been missing in action and largely absent, or whether you've experienced something in between, having a baby exposes all the weak spots in any couple relationship, and you're bound to have had some moments of feeling disconnected as a couple since the baby arrived. Though it's normal to feel this way, focusing on that thought—that he's *doing it wrong* by not understanding what you're going through as a new mom, not helping out enough, siding with his mother in criticism of your parenting choices (or not stepping in to defend you), or whatever the case may be—will inevitably cause stress and conflict.

Consider this scenario:

> *You and your husband come home from another long day at the office. You're both delighted to see the baby and spend time with her, but someone has to empty the dishwasher, get dinner, pay the bills, call the guy to repair the dryer, and take out the trash. Knowing that he won't take the initiative on any of these, you whip through the to-do list while he plays with the baby and turns on the news, killing him softly in your mind.*

Some of you mamas reading these words might be tempted to label this dad a slacker, and maybe he is. But even more important is how judging your husband makes you feel. Calm or stressed? Connected to him or disconnected? Angry or loving? The answer to these is pretty obvious. Rather than blaming him, you could:

- **Cancel negative thoughts,** dropping the blame—*He does whatever he wants, never thinking about my needs,* for instance. It's really as simple as just making the choice to let go. Take a deep breath in, and on the exhale breath, just release all negative thoughts about this man who helped you bring your precious baby into the world.

- **Allow your feelings.** Go ahead and register the physical sensations of anger, annoyance, hurt, or whatever other emotions may be present—maybe a prickly feeling on your neck, a throbbing sensation behind your eyes, or a ball of slimy green goo in your stomach. Just witness what you feel, without reacting or commentary, as you come all the way into your body. Take another deep breath. If it helps, say your truth out loud: "I'm feeling *really,* incredibly, unbelievably annoyed."

- **Link up and listen.** Tough one—but worth it, as connecting with your husband and understanding his point of view may prevent you from having an unnecessary argument. Whether you decide to have a conversation now or later, when you do talk, step into his shoes for a moment so you can see his perspective, then *listen.* Here's what you might find:

  - Maybe he'd just like to have a little bit of downtime before going through the to-do list.

  - Maybe he's so used to you taking charge of all that there is "to do" that he's decided to stay out of your way.

  - As he's talking, you might find your own reflection in the mirror as you discover that you rarely, if ever, let yourself have downtime, constantly pushing yourself to stay on task with taking care of the baby, whatever work you bring home, and the household instead. Translation: your husband is better at taking care of himself than you are at taking care of yourself.

- **Mirror.** As you gather information, reflect back to him what you're hearing and intuiting. Remember, you're not working on solutions yet, and you'll have a chance to express whatever you need to in just another moment.

- "You really want to relax for a few minutes at the end of a long day before diving into all there is to do. Who doesn't?"
- "So to you, it feels like I've been giving you a mixed message. I want to be in charge, but then I complain about you not helping more."
- "I get that you're not sure what I need, because I haven't really been clear about that."

By the time you get to the end of these steps, you'll often find that you feel much more relaxed—your body says, *Ahhhh.* That's your signal that you've truly connected both with yourself and him; the connection itself will now carry you to whatever other steps you may wish to take toward resolution.

If this was a common theme in your relationship—where you felt like you were picking up way more of the slack (and let's face it, division of labor is a common theme of conflict for many parents)—you may now want to speak up about that, though ideally you would have this conversation at a time when you could both focus, such as after the baby was sleeping or on a weekend. Having already taken the time to connect, the likelihood of having a peaceful, productive conversation would be exponentially higher than if you had not. At whatever point you decided to have that conversation, you could continue to cycle through the steps for CALM—perhaps also using your anchor and the Calming Breath exercise—to help communication flow as smoothly as possible.

Love Makes the World Go 'Round

Derek often does an interesting exercise in his workshops, and it goes like this: on a scale from 1 to 10, pick a number that describes how much you love yourself—1 is loving yourself a little, while 10 is loving yourself so much that if you were a giant ice cream cone, you'd lick yourself to death! Just go with the first number that pops into your head.

Here's how to score: If you gave yourself somewhere between a 1 and a 4, your self-esteem is fairly low. If you're between a 5 and a 7, you're in the majority—you like some qualities about yourself well enough but still see plenty of room for improvement. If you gave yourself a 7 to 9, well done! You have fairly healthy self-esteem. And if you gave yourself a 10, well, your husband is one lucky guy, because someone who loves herself that unconditionally is capable of loving others unconditionally, too. And that's the point of this exercise; your number reflects the level to which you're able to give to others, because we can only love another to the extent that we love ourselves.

So if you gave yourself a 6, guess what? You are capable of loving your significant other only a 6. That's not to say that you aren't capable of lavishing him with plenty of affection and care, but if his wishes and needs are greater than 6 on a 10 scale, that's going to cause some friction between you. Now here's the other part of the equation: If you're a 6, you're capable of *receiving* love only to a 6 as well. Believe it or not, if more than that were offered, you either wouldn't recognize it or you would unconsciously reject it and push it away. The good news is that your number isn't fixed; you can change it by practicing more self-acceptance.

By the way, babies don't only mirror back your unclaimed negativity; they also mirror back your unclaimed *love*. When your baby adores you and that feels overwhelming or provokes anxiety in you, it may be because she loves you more than you love yourself.

My Parents/In-Laws/ Relatives Are Doing It Wrong

In Chapter 5, we talked about the dangers of giving too much power to all of the people in your orbit who may have opinions and advice, solicited or unsolicited, about the best ways to parent a baby and raise a child. Making any of them the "bad guy," though, is an equally slippery slope. Let's take a grandparent, for instance. Let's say that every time your mom visits, she brings a truckload of toys and gadgets, though you've asked her not to do that. Or maybe she grabs the baby out of your arms, greeting her with a loud, animated voice: "*Hi, baby!*" she says, then proceeds to tickle, squeeze, and bounce the baby for the entire visit. It isn't long before the baby begins to melt down, what with all that input into her not-yet-developed sensory system.

Or how about this scenario: your husband didn't get the promotion you both thought he would, and your combined salaries barely stretch you to making ends meet since the baby's arrival. Despite knowing this, your financially stable in-laws decline your request for assistance. Or try this one: your sister-in-law, who has older kids of her own, acts like a know-it-all, offering advice on your every move as a parent. "If you hold her all day long, she'll come to expect that," she might admonish. When you tell her that you have the baby sleeping in your room with you, she's horrified: "You've got to get her out of there," she insists. "You'll never sleep, and you'll never have sex, and the next thing you know your marriage will tank. Trust me."

For better and worse, there will be loved ones in your orbit—grandparents, aunts, siblings, cousins, friends—who say and do all kinds of things that drive you nuts. Some of it will be mildly annoying; some of it will trigger you more strongly. If it feels like you're being attacked, your brain (in fight-flight-freeze mode) will argue with you that you should turn away, defend, or strike out, so deciding not to react can sometimes feel superhuman, especially if what's happening (the criticism, the feeling that you're being steamrollered) is a familiar pattern in the relationship. Here's how CALM can help.

> For better and worse, there will be loved ones in your orbit—grandparents, aunts, siblings, cousins, friends— who say and do all kinds of things that drive you nuts.

- **Cancel negative thoughts.** Even if your mother-in-law is criticizing your choice to bottle feed/cosleep with the baby/ go back to work *yet again*, putting her in the bad guy position will only make you feel worse—and more stressed. Take a deep breath, reminding yourself that she is who she is, and exhale.

- **Allow your feelings.** Rather than shutting down or reacting with lots of emotion, come all the way into your body: feel your feet on the ground, and notice the sensations you feel. If you're registering hurt or anger, see where you are feeling these emotions—chest, stomach, shoulders?—and describe to yourself in detail what they feel like. Take another deep breath; breathing deeply will help you counterbalance the stress hormones that are flooding through your body.

- **Link up and listen.** No matter what it seems like, someone who is attacking and criticizing feels threatened or vulnerable in some way. If you choose not to react but to connect instead, taking a moment to better understand where your mother-in-law is coming from, you'll help diffuse a potential negative reaction. You can ask why she disagrees with your choice or just tune in within, using all of your senses and your intuition, to gather information. All kinds of possibilities may pop up:

  - She explains that she was a working mom herself and feels guilty about not being there for her own kids.

  - You remember that she was a stay-at-home mom who always wished she could have a career, and you realize that she may be feeling some envy.

  - She strongly encouraged her own children toward independence, and your practice of cosleeping may feel threatening to that choice.

  The idea here is not to agree with what she's saying, necessarily, or to affirm your hypotheses as facts, but rather to "try on" her perspective so you can depersonalize her attack.

- **Mirror.** Resist the urge to defend yourself, and instead reflect back to her your best interpretation of what you've picked up on as you connected and listened.

  - "I know going back to work isn't the choice you would have made. Staying home with your kids was really right for you."

  - "You feel very strongly about this subject. That's really clear!"

  - "Cosleeping wasn't a common practice when your kids were babies. I'm sure it's hard to imagine since you haven't experienced it."

You might find that after moving through these steps, you feel fairly relaxed; the emotional charge isn't nearly as strong, and no further action is necessary. On the other hand, you may feel inclined to speak up: "We're actually really happy with the choice we've made about [breastfeeding, cosleeping, my going back to work]—it's something we've thought about a lot, and it's working out well for us." Whatever you're guided to do or say, go for it! You can feel confident knowing that you'll be doing so from a much calmer place than would be the case if you had succumbed to emotional reactivity.

By the way, as you read through the steps for CALM during challenges that arise with others, it may seem like getting to *But what do I do?!* is taking forever. You may want to reconsider the idea that there's always something to *do* when big feelings arise; sometimes the "doing" is more about staying present and centered in your body than taking any outward action. You may find, more often than not, that what comes next (if anything) happens quite naturally.

When big feelings arise, sometimes the "doing" is more about staying present and centered in your body than taking any outward action.

The Importance of Listening

When you're having a difficult exchange with someone, notice that when you start to check out of your body and disconnect, you also stop listening to the other person and start listening to your own self-talk instead: all the reasons why you're right and they're wrong. When you're holding connection with the other person as the priority, on the other hand, listening becomes a higher priority, too. Throughout your day, practice listening and mirroring with others as often as you can; developing this muscle will help you do so more easily in the heat of conflict, when your resistance will come up strongly.

My Child Is Doing It Wrong

Some of you, especially if you have a baby younger than six months, might believe that this is a mama mantra you would *never* entertain. Others of you, on the other hand, may find that you're feeling irritable throughout your day as a mom, or frustrated that your baby isn't sleeping or feeding well (especially if you've worked hard on these things), or overwhelmed by her clinginess if she's hit a new developmental phase, for example. This mama mantra can also pop up when you haven't been taking enough time for yourself recently. When you are focused on your child and her needs all day long, it can feel like there's little room for you. And as much as you may enjoy spending time together, if *all* you're doing is dangling toys, singing "Twinkle Twinkle, Little Star," and feeding, burping, and changing her, you may start to feel a bit stir crazy—or just plain crazy. Any of these can indicate a possible imbalance in the relationship that could use some adjusting.

The other thing that can happen is that once you pass through the newborn phase and your child's personality begins to emerge—usually beginning at about six to nine months, and really kicking in once your child heads toward toddlerhood—her will starts to assert itself, and your baby can suddenly seem defiant or, if she's well into toddler territory, like she's grown three heads. *Who is this little monster*, you might think, *and what has she done with my sweet, innocent angel?*

Remember in Chapter 5 how we talked about the idea that if you have a tendency to want to control things, you likely felt overly responsible for one or both of your parents growing up? Well, there's a flip side: reacting to being controlled. If this is a button for you, you may have a history of feeling that you had to give up control in a relationship with one or both parents in order to be loved. You may have had needs that you didn't often express—believing that a response wasn't possible or likely—or you may have found that when you did speak up, you got in trouble or were dismissed. Today, with your child, it may similarly feel as though there's no room for your needs in the relationship, and that it's all about her instead. In frustration, you may blame or criticize your child, mistakenly believing that she's got all the control or that she should be able to meet your needs, such as to sleep, eat, or behave as consistently as you'd like her to (which isn't possible).

See if any of these statements sound familiar:

- *My child is unusually challenging and strong-willed.*
- *My child knows just how to push all of my buttons— and create new ones.*

- *It feels like my child is determined to make my life miserable.*

- *My child won't listen to me and won't behave the way I need her to.*

- *I'm often embarrassed by my child's crying or acting-out behavior.*

- *My child is too needy. I give and give, and she always wants more.*

- *I often have highly charged reactions to my child's behavior.*

- *I feel frustrated that my child _____ (fill in the blank).*

- *When someone criticizes my parenting choices, I get angry.*

- *I often feel drained, irritable, frustrated, angry, and resentful as a mom.*

The common sentiment in these statements is, *I've made my child responsible for my happiness.* On some level, you believe that your child has all the power, and that leads to resentment about feeling controlled.

Some moms find that they have more of a tendency to *reach for control* in the first twelve months or so of a child's life, when the baby's needs are relatively straightforward, and then begin to feel resentment about *feeling controlled* by their child's willfulness once she starts to test limits. Consider this scenario:

AJ is feeding lunch to her baby, Maddie, ten months; on Maddie's high-chair tray are some chicken and pasta shells and her sippy cup. After taking a sip of water, she drops her cup on the floor. "Oopsie!" AJ says cheerfully, picking it up for her and putting it back on the tray. Moments later, and looking right at AJ, Maddie pushes a few

shells over the side of the tray. AJ picks those up, too, albeit a little
less cheerfully this time. Over the next several minutes, Maddie drops
her cup on the floor three more times, plus some chicken too; she's
relishing the game with glee. Exasperated, AJ decides that lunchtime
is over, and Maddie proceeds to throw a fit.

Part of the task for any mom and baby, as the baby grows and your relationship moves forward, is for you to accept both the positive *and* negative traits in each other—and we all have a combination of both, even your baby. A large part of the focus of this book has been about accepting all that you are—the good, the bad, and the ugly; in doing so, you are much better equipped to accept both the good and not-so-good traits in your baby, your husband or partner, and everyone else in your orbit, too. The baby's developmental task is to do the same for you; as she grows, from her perspective you go from the all-good mommy who meets her needs to the sometimes-bad mommy who sometimes doesn't, and as she starts to move toward toddlerhood, she's probably going to have some pretty strong feelings about that. Your task as the mom is to tolerate her projections, as well as your own ups and downs about your child's emotions and behavior, by staying as nonreactive as you can. As you communicate to your baby that you can tolerate all the different parts of her, she continues to feel safe in the relationship and maintains positive self-esteem. (Note that your baby will need discipline at times, of course; it's perfectly okay, and important, to set healthy limits with her when appropriate.)

You can absolutely work with CALM to stay centered during challenging interactions with your child. Scenarios like these are also good opportunities to use your anchor and breathe deeply, perhaps incorporating the Calming Breath exercise. But there's another opportunity here as well: to look in the mirror. If you're repeatedly feeling a strong charge—6 and above on a 1 to 10 scale—about a particular behavior that your child is doing, she may be bringing to light something in yourself that you haven't fully addressed. In the example of the scenario above, if AJ felt *very* strong feelings about Maddie's limit-testing behavior, Maddie could be mirroring:

> As you communicate to your baby that you can tolerate all the different parts of her, she continues to feel safe in the relationship and maintains positive self-esteem.

- AJ's own defiant behavior, such as when her husband tells her repeatedly that he doesn't feel it's a good time to buy a new house, but she keeps pushing anyway;

- AJ's defiant behavior from once upon a time, for instance when she was a teenager, which she may look back on with shame or self-blame; or

- AJ's *timid* behavior, which is the flipside of defiance; perhaps she rarely speaks up for herself or expresses her own needs, and seeing this behavior in Maddie is making her uncomfortable.

These are just ideas. If it feels difficult to recognize yourself in the mirror of behavior in your child that triggers you often, try focusing on the emotion you're feeling, and see if a movie from the past pops up in your theater that gives you some clues.

Professionals and Other "Experts" Are Doing It Wrong

As we talked about in Chapter 5, doctors, parenting professionals, and so-called parenting experts sometimes do have valuable information or wisdom to offer—and sometimes they get it wrong. Consider this scenario:

> *Theresa has been caregiver to Stella, six months, since her birth. One day Jackie, Stella's mom, notices that Stella's head seems unusually flat in the back, but Theresa, who's been working with children for twenty years, insists it's nothing to worry about. A month later, Jackie brings Stella to the doctor for an ear infection, and the doctor diagnoses Stella with plagiocephaly— "flat head" —explaining that Stella will likely need to wear a helmet for several months. Jackie is livid.*

Although Jackie's anger at Theresa is understandable, looking at this scenario objectively, can you see how her inclination to blame Theresa for "doing it wrong"—suggesting that Stella's flat head was nothing to worry about—is really misplaced anger at *herself* for not following her own instincts that there was something amiss? We've noticed that often when a mom becomes angry with someone in her orbit she's turned to for advice and the advice doesn't pan out well for her or her baby, she sensed that the advice was a little off but followed it anyway, trusting that the person with more experience must know best. Now, sometimes you'll have those little niggling doubts about a piece of parenting guidance and everything turns out just fine when you follow it and your concern turns out to be unfounded; conversely, sometimes you won't get any red flags, but following the advice doesn't take you to the result you'd hoped for. The problem isn't actually in taking a leap of faith to follow someone else's advice; rather, it's in giving someone else the credit or the blame for what happens next. If you decide to follow outside advice, *you* are the one making that choice; no one is forcing you to do that. So if the net result turns out favorably, that's great! And if it doesn't, you'll have learned something valuable and gained even more wisdom about what's best for your baby.

> The problem isn't in taking a leap of faith to follow someone else's advice; rather, it's in giving someone else the credit or the blame for what happens next.

If you receive guidance from a professional that impacts the baby in a serious way—for instance, a doctor misdiagnoses or mistreats a medical condition—then you'll want to address the situation of course, though working with CALM or one of the other supports in Chapter 3 can help you do so from a centered place that's based in empowerment rather than in lots of emotion and reactivity.

Everybody Else Is Wrong

When you become a mom, you suddenly become much more invested in what the people around you are and are not doing, as their actions could potentially affect your baby's well-being. What this means is that just about everyone becomes a potential suspect in the ongoing trial called *My Baby's Well-being vs. the World:*

- the neighbor who mows his lawn in the middle of the baby's nap
- the person who drives by on a loud motorcycle and frightens the baby
- the mom friend who mistakenly told you that you could keep breastmilk in the fridge for a week
- the sales clerk who forgot to put the diaper wipes in your grocery bag
- the baby in your mommy class who keeps crawling over to your baby and grabbing her hair
- your supervisor at work, who declines your request to take another month before returning

People are people, and they do what they do. When they throw a wrench into your baby's day, or yours, pause—and breathe—before doing anything else.

Taking Personal Responsibility for Your Happiness and Well-Being

The cast of characters in this chapter are a motley crew of individuals who may or may not be considering your best interests, or your baby's. They will inevitably push your buttons, make you see red, bring up your stuff, steamroller over your authority as a mom, and criticize your parenting choices. Think about it this way: Each of these encounters gives you yet another opportunity to practice responding rather than reacting. Each time you do, you'll become an even stronger mom.

Looking in the Mirror

When another person triggers you, notice what you think and feel, and what happens in your body. Because you are seeing yourself in a mirror, these reactions are like a map that can help you understand yourself better. Take a look at the typical thoughts, feelings, and reactions that arise when you interact with:

- your baby (and other children if you have more than one)

- your husband or partner

- your mother

- your father

- your mother-in-law and/or father-in-law

- your caregiver

- your supervisor at work

- your close friends

- your pediatrician

- yourself, when you're alone (and if you're *never* alone, take a look at that, too!)

CHAPTER 7

Negative
Mama Mantra No. 3:
Things Went Wrong
in the Past or Will Go
Wrong in the Future

How Getting Stuck
in the Past and Projecting into
the Future Cause **Stress**

Ihere is only one thing we can say, unequivocally, about the past: it can't be changed. If we could accept this truth fully, we wouldn't need therapists or self-help books, we wouldn't get addicted to anything, and there would be no broken-hearted love songs about not being able to get over an old flame. If we didn't dwell on the past, we'd certainly be a whole lot happier, and we'd have a lot more energy to boot. Best of all, we would simply forgive others for perceived wrongs, permanently wiping out the scorecard we each keep about the hurts we've incurred, and we'd forgive ourselves, too, for any wrongs we felt we'd committed. Imagine feeling that liberated!

What an ominous task you have as a mom: not only is it your job to take care of your child 24-7—getting her to sleep, making sure she eats her veggies, tending to her "owies" as she explores her world, offering a hug or some encouragement when she needs it—but interacting with her brings up your stuff *all the time*. Example: When your baby cries, it feels like someone is hanging you upside down by your toenails. Or when she'll neither eat the dinner you made her on her own nor let you feed it to her, you feel more than a little annoyed. These kinds of reactions go well beyond the normal emotional ups and downs that any parent feels on a daily basis, and every parent has these buttons, whether a few or dozens. When they get pushed—causing a strong emotional charge of anger, sadness, or anxiety in you—what's actually happening is that current events are lighting up old familiar neural pathways, thanks to the memories, conscious or unconscious, that your child is triggering. In other words, the projectionist in your internal theater is busily queuing up movies, and your adult self in the here and now and your child self from the past are both having an emotional reaction simultaneously. What fun!

When your buttons get pushed, current events are lighting up old neural pathways.

If you're like most parents, when strong emotions arise you'll do your best to avoid them or push them back down; you've got a baby to take care of and a busy life, and who has time to deal with feelings? And yet, as we've been discussing throughout this book, avoiding your feelings will almost certainly cause stress and anxiety for you, which will then have a trickle-down effect on your little bright light, affecting her mood and behavior, too. Sometimes when the baby is fussing, you may try to hold her, offer the breast or bottle, or rock, bounce, or swing her in response—and yet she still fusses anyway. Or you may experiment with some tried-and-true baby-calming techniques, and sometimes, maybe even often, those handy tricks will work. But sometimes they won't. And some of *those* times, the reason you can't settle your baby is that you yourself feel unsettled and completely split in two. You're supposed to be the grown-up, the adult, the *mom*; you're supposed to attend to your baby and comfort her. But because the baby in your arms is triggering all kinds of emotions in you, you've got what seems like an impossible dilemma: How can you be a calm mama when you feel so overwhelmed?

Getting Stuck in the Past

Most of us don't fully come face-to-face with the past until we bump up against it in the context of an adult relationship. You probably met some of the wounded parts of yourself in your dating life, and they may have popped up in other relationships, too. They're the ones who cause you to act like a five-year-old who throws a tantrum when she isn't getting needs met, or who feels terribly victimized and pouts when hurt, or who shrinks and shuts down when afraid—even if you're usually a fairly even-tempered person. In fact, you're probably still contending with some of these patterns in your relationship with the baby's other parent (who, by the way, also has his own wounds, of course). But some parts of yourself that emerged when you became a mother may have remained well hidden until that point, because you'd never been a parent before. As we've said, this is partly why parenting is so intense; painful experiences from the past, some of which date back many years, are suddenly back to revisit you, along with all of the emotions you *didn't* get to fully process the first time around because you didn't have the tools to do so back then. The more challenging your childhood experiences, of course, the more painful the feelings and memories surrounding them can be; this is often why the postpartum emotional experience can feel so much more difficult for one mom than another.

> For better and worse, part of being a parent is coming to terms with the past—and whatever emotions, painful or pleasant, hop along for the ride.

And so, for better and worse, part of being a parent is coming to terms with the past—and whatever emotions, painful or pleasant, hop along for the ride. It's not always easy to show up for what you're feeling, but the alternative is trying to carry on being a mom when feeling emotionally disconnected, which can make for a much more challenging parenting experience. In other words, not attending to what's going on inside of you is not exactly the easy way out; if anything, it's the tougher road to travel. You've likely already discovered this for yourself. Whether you feel like you are riding the waves of your emotional experience as a mom fairly well, whether you spend every waking moment feeling seasick from all the turbulence, or whether you fall somewhere in between is not a report card that evaluates your fitness for being a parent, nor is it a reflection on who you are as a person. But every mom can benefit from learning how to become a better surfer.

Discovering Emotional Triggers

If you feel strong emotions (lots of anxiety, sadness, or anger) on a regular basis when a certain scenario or behavior pattern surfaces with your child, you can be pretty certain that your past is informing your present. Don't shoot the messenger: these feelings are pointing toward places in your childhood where you experienced emotional discon- nection from a trusted adult (likely a parent) as well as yourself, and because similar emotions are coming up now, you have an opportunity to repair those disconnections. On a 1 to 10 scale, 10 being "I'm feeling a really strong feeling," if you register 5 and above on any of the below on a regular basis, these may be emotional triggers for you.

- Your baby cries for any reason.
- Your child struggles—learning how to roll or crawl, or trying to figure out how to interact with a new toy.
- Your child seems to prefer the other parent to you.
- Your child dissolves into a puddle of tears and apparent helplessness when frustrated.
- Your child is incredibly sensitive, crying loudly when getting her diaper changed or getting dressed, when hungry, or when riding in the car.
- Your child acts like Velcro—she can't tolerate separation from you.
- Your child reacts negatively to deviations from the normal routine.

> • Your growing baby tests limits: you tell her "no," and she goes ahead anyway.
>
> Remember, as far as the amygdala is concerned, the past deeply informs the present. If you're regularly feeling either disconnected from your emotions or highly reactive during certain kinds of interaction with your child, there's a good chance that your internal theater is playing old home movies while current events are unfolding.

Dealing with Emotional Triggers

What a cruel irony: you can't change the past, but as a parent the past seems very much alive in the present through your child. And for that reason, you can't help feeling the feelings that get triggered in your interactions with her. But what if that cruel irony is actually an incredible gift? Consider this: *because* your past is coming up now in the mirror of your child, you have a golden opportunity to reconnect with a part of you that is stuck in the past and to heal old wounds.

Emotional triggers happen unconsciously; you can't help your buttons getting pushed and the feelings arising, and when this happens, your tendency may be to ignore or avoid what you're feeling because it's painful. That doesn't work, of course—though who hasn't tried it? What's more, disconnecting from yourself this way and denying your feelings allows all of that unclaimed emotion, and resulting stress, to flow right on through the invisible umbilical to your child. Without having your example of what it looks like to feel and manage emotions, she may develop the same tendency to ignore, suppress, or distract herself from her own feelings as she continues to grow, too.

It's Okay to Show Your Emotions

You do *not* have to act calm and happy around your baby all the time. It's perfectly okay to allow the baby to witness you feeling emotions like sadness or frustration, as this teaches her what emotions are and how to manage them. For example, you can say, "I'm so frustrated that we got a parking ticket! I'm going to take a few deep breaths to calm down before we start driving." Talking about what you're feeling, and modeling how you handle your emotions, teaches her how to regulate her own emotions, too.

If you feel a bit lost when it comes to dealing with emotions, you're not alone. Most of us grew up with parents who didn't always know how to tolerate their own feelings very well, so they didn't know how to teach us how to do that, either; instead, many of us got messages that what we were feeling wasn't welcome or convenient, so we learned to shut our feelings down. Now that you're a parent yourself, you may know that it's healthy to feel your emotions and to allow your child to feel her feelings, too, but you may have little or no idea about how to do either of these. That's okay, it's never too late to learn—and it's also perfectly fine to learn right alongside your child. CALM can help.

If you feel a bit lost when it comes to dealing with emotions, you're not alone.

When you stay present with your emotions as they surface, you not only experience the benefits of connecting with yourself in the here and now—which often include feeling much more calm and centered as feelings move through you rather than staying stuck—but you also connect with that past part of you who didn't have anyone to connect with when she felt those intense feelings the first time around, and who probably felt pretty overwhelmed as a result. Though the charge may feel intense briefly as emotions start to come up, it usually also dissipates fairly quickly, often in a matter of seconds if you stay present rather than check out; as a happy side benefit, once you allow your emotions to express, you're much less likely to be triggered in similar circumstances going forward. This is because each time you allow your emotions to arise rather than shoving them aside or stuffing them down, the child inside of you grows up a bit. It's not necessary to relive the specifics of old pain and trauma; simply honoring your feelings by staying present with them in the here and now is enough to change the way you navigate your overall emotional landscape.

What about a new mom's shifting hormones—don't those strongly influence emotions, too? Indeed they do, though mounting research on the mind-body connection indicates that our thoughts can produce all kinds of physiological responses, influencing our health and well-being. Science shows us that whatever we think, our cells will agree; even when you're not aware of your thoughts, your body is listening.[18] What the mind believes, it achieves.

Dealing with Anxiety

Anxiety can be connected to the idea that something that's happening shouldn't be, or that you're "doing it wrong." It can also spike sharply when the brain connects current events to past painful memories or when you're worried about your baby's well-being. Consider this scenario:

> *Every time her baby, Jake, cries, Emma feels like there is broken glass coursing through her veins. Panic rises up inside of her, and she quickly picks up the baby to do whatever it takes—rocking, bouncing, shushing, feeding—to help him (and herself) settle. When Jake cries, it feels to Emma like she herself is in danger or crisis, and that something bad will happen if she doesn't make him stop.*

What Emma is experiencing is far beyond the normal sense of urgency that most moms feel when their baby cries. She is feeling strong fear, and stress hormones in her body are triggering fight-flight-freeze. When you find yourself feeling a much stronger emotion than a situation warrants—for instance, you constantly worry that your child isn't okay (i.e., something is *wrong*), despite all evidence to the contrary—that's a surefire sign that a painful dynamic from your past, probably with a parent, is being triggered. You don't actually need to know the specifics of what that trigger is about, nor do you need to analyze it. Instead, your task is simply to attend to your feelings rather than avoid them.

Here's how Emma could do that by working with CALM. As soon as Jake started to cry, she would:

- **Cancel negative thoughts.** When Jake cries, Emma might be thinking something like, *I can't stand the baby's crying, and he needs to stop* or, if she blamed herself for not being able to "fix" it for him, *Why can't I stop him from crying?* Emma would take a big, deep breath and let go of those thoughts on her exhale.

- **Allow her feelings.** Emma would then acknowledge that she was feeling anxious and turn her attention to the physical sensations of that emotion in her body, perhaps the throbbing of her pulse in her temples, the tightness in her forearms and shoulders, the tension in her brows and jaw, and the sharp, shooting pangs in her stomach. She would take another deep breath, or several, right into the places where she felt tense energy or anxiety.

- **Link up and listen.** Emma would then connect with Jake through the invisible umbilical, sharing her love, listening, and gathering information about what he was experiencing (perhaps the sound of crying but no actual tears, a halfhearted, tired-sounding wail, and some head movement but no other visible agitation).

- **Mirror.** Emma would reflect whatever she noticed back to Jake, perhaps something like: "You're crying, but you're not super upset. Even though you're fussing, there aren't actually any tears. You're just grumbling a bit, and you might be tired because you took a short nap. Mommy's right here with you, sweetie. I see your body starting to relax a bit now."

Emma might be surprised to find that as she focused her calm attention on Jake, he began to calm, too, as he felt his mama connecting with him. On the other hand, if Emma noticed that she was still feeling anxiety in her body, or if Jake did start to become more upset, she could move through the steps again.

Remember, the steps for CALM may not always seem linear when you're in the moment; for example, Emma might have begun to focus on the sensations in her body and then remembered to cancel her negative thoughts. The order in which you do the steps, and how long you spend on each one, is entirely up to you. Don't let yourself leapfrog over allowing your feelings, though!

I'll Be There

When strong emotions are present, the message *I'm right here with you*, whether communicating that sentiment to your baby, another person, or yourself, is a very powerful one. The truth is that most of us don't actually want or need anyone to fix or change our experiences for us, even the painful ones; what we really want instead is simply for someone to keep us company while we're having them. That's good to remember when you or your baby seems upset or uncomfortable.

Dealing with Sadness

Sadness is another common emotion for moms, and it can pop up when you least expect it—when you're tired, when there's conflict with your husband, and even when you're feeding your baby, particularly if you're recalling (consciously or not) a feeling of not being attended to in the way you would have liked as a child. Let's take a look at what happens when this is the primary emotion being triggered.

Georgia, mom to one-month-old Christopher, sometimes feels an overwhelming sense of sadness when she is holding her baby. When she gazes at him, even though she's feeling lots of love, her heart feels heavy, too, and the tears just flow. Georgia has no idea why she feels this way.

Working with CALM, Georgia would:

- <u>C</u>ancel negative thoughts she might be having, such as *I shouldn't be feeling this way* (I'm doing it wrong), *I can't let Christopher see me cry* (I'm doing it wrong again), or any version of *Something was wrong in the past,* which could be coming up if there was an old movie playing in her internal theater.

- <u>A</u>llow her feelings. Even if she was holding Christopher, Georgia could notice where in her body she was feeling sadness. She would describe the feeling to herself in as much detail as possible, asking questions like these:
  - What color is this sadness?
  - What shape does it have?
  - Is it moving or staying still?
  - Are the edges blurry or clear?
  - Is it hot or cold? Heavy or light?

  Georgia would then take several more deep breaths right into the places where she was feeling the highest concentration of emotion in her body. She might remind herself, *It's perfectly okay for this sadness to be here.*

- <u>L</u>ink up and listen. Even though Christopher himself may not be crying or needing attention, Georgia would connect with him anyway, sharing her love and tuning in. She might notice the calm and peaceful expression on his face, or the way his fingers curled and uncurled around her own. She might pay attention to his soft vocalizations, and to the steady rhythms of his breathing. Connecting with Christopher this way would help Georgia to stay in the present moment.

- <u>M</u>irror. Georgia could then mirror back to Christopher what she was noticing, either out loud or silently:

  - "You're so peaceful right now."

  - "You're looking up at Mommy, and it's so nice just to be here together."

  - "I really treasure these moments with you."

Georgia could also talk to Christopher about her tears, if she was having them, saying something like, "Mommy's crying because I feel sad right now. I don't know why I feel sad, but I'm taking care of myself by letting my tears come. I love you very much." Remember, though you aren't trying to figure out why you feel the way you feel as you move through the steps, insights about that might pop up. If they do, just let them come.

Don't Be Afraid to Ask for Help

If you have a history of childhood trauma, if you and/or the baby experienced trauma during pregnancy or delivery, if your child has had a serious medical issue, or if there are other family stressors, such as financial worries or having an extended family member with an illness, you may feel strong emotion on a regular basis, or conversely feelings of numbness. If it feels too overwhelming to manage your emotions on your own, enlist the support of a trusted loved one or a professional who can assist you.

Dealing with Anger

Some moms don't feel much of this emotion until their baby is old enough to test limits, usually somewhere between nine and twelve months. Other moms may feel surges of anger or resentment much earlier, such as when the baby refuses to nap or constantly demands your attention, or when life as a mom just feels hard. Anger comes when you have a desire that's not being fulfilled; for a mom, that desire can revolve around anything from wanting the baby to wake up later in the morning and eat more veggies to wishing she would play more independently or go with the flow a bit more. Consider this scenario:

To Carolyn, everything with eleven-month-old Ava suddenly feels like a battle. Ava hates getting her diaper changed, puts up a big stink when it's time to get out of the bath, and fights Carolyn when getting into her car seat. Ava also has a big reaction when Carolyn tells her no, such as when she's trying to play with the phone or dump out the table salt at a restaurant. Carolyn's anger spikes up all throughout the day, like mercury in a thermometer.

In addition to CALM, there are several other supports from Chapter 3 that might work well here; one would be to do lots of deep breathing, perhaps focusing particularly on the Calming Breath exercise. Another would be to work with the Grounding exercise; staying focused in the body can be particularly challenging when anger is spiking. Working with the Heart of Gold meditation on a regular basis could also help prevent anger from spiking during more stressful moments with the baby. Lastly, Carolyn might Tune In Within to access clear guidance about how to best handle Ava's testing and tantrums.

Editing Your Old Home Movies

If you were a child who didn't feel safe allowing and expressing her feelings, allowing your feelings to surface now as a parent may feel unfamiliar and uncomfortable at first. Please know that this is common. Your baby is actually an excellent teacher on this subject: watch as she expresses intense upset one minute, then laughs with delight the next. Emotions are supposed to be fluid; they are meant to come and go quickly—ninety seconds, to be exact—not to stay stuck inside of us for weeks, months, or years.

As a new mom, it's normal for your emotions to feel overwhelming at times. That's partly about the love you have for your baby— everything is heightened because you are so

As a new mom, it's normal for your emotions to feel overwhelming at times.

invested in her care and well-being—and partly about discovering pockets of emotion that have been pent up inside of you since you were a child. All any of us really want when we're having big emotions is for someone to be present with us while we're having them. That person may at times be your spouse, your mother, or your best friend, but you don't want to be dependent on an outside source who might not always be available. If *you* can learn how to be present with yourself while experiencing your emotions, whatever additional support you may receive will only build on what you're already giving to yourself, in a positive way. As you allow yourself to feel your feelings, you'll become more adept at riding their waves rather than getting drowned by them. As a bonus, your child benefits and learns by watching you. As you choose to stay present with your emotions, you are effectively taking one of your old movies into the editing room and creating an entirely new cinematic experience, connecting with yourself to repair a prior emotional disconnect; in other words, you are rewiring neural pathways. Over time, those old pathways—painful emotional triggers and habits of avoiding or denying your feelings altogether—begin to shrink from underuse as you choose the path of accepting your emotions instead.

Stressful situations in which strong feelings come up are like little mini-classes that teach you something valuable.

Remember, too, that difficult situations and stress are not the enemy; when these do come along, you have an opportunity to put into practice new skills that you are learning. From that perspective, stressful situations in which strong feelings come up are like little mini-classes that teach you something valuable. If you are going to be a teacher for your baby, then you also have to be willing to be the student sometimes, too. That doesn't mean that you

are letting your baby down—far from it! By showing her that you are
still learning yourself, you can illustrate an important truth: that life
is always our teacher, and there are always new opportunities to learn
and grow. She, too, will have her share of stressful situations as she
graduates from baby and toddler to child, teen, and adult—and with
your example, she'll have lots of healthy options for how to handle
her own emotions along the way.

Using CALM to Manage Emotions

Sometimes your feelings may come up so strongly that the *Allow
your feelings* step in CALM doesn't give you quite enough time to
process them fully. When this happens, and when your baby doesn't
need immediate attention, you can cycle through all of the steps for
CALM focusing just on you instead. Here's how.

- **Cancel negative thoughts.** If you're not used to staying present with strong emotions, thoughts like, *I shouldn't feel this
  way* or, *It's pointless to get angry* or, *I can't handle feeling
  sad* might pop up. Your mind doesn't want you to feel your
  feelings, because then it would out of a job! Just take a big,
  deep breath, and on your exhale breath, let all those negative
  thoughts release. If they pop up again at any point during
  the rest of the steps, just use your breath to release them in
  the same way.

- **Allow your feelings.** This may be the opposite of what you
  feel like doing. Because your brain will be registering fear,
  and thus triggering fight-flight-freeze, you may be tempted
  to shut down or check out. Instead, get into your body and

get specific on the physical sensations of the emotion you're feeling. Focusing on the details of what you're experiencing will help you stay present. Ask yourself:

- *What emotion am I feeling primarily?* (If it's tough to get a specific read, start with the big three: anxiety, sadness, anger.)

- *Where is this feeling in my body?* (i.e., head, stomach, throat, hips, hands). Now describe the feeling in as much detail as possible: *What shape is it? What color is it? Is it moving or staying still? Is it hot or cold? Are the edges blurry or clear? Is it heavy or light? Is there anything that this feeling wants to say?*

- <u>**Link up and listen.**</u> Connect—this time with yourself—and listen to the answers you get to the questions in the prior step, for instance, *I'm feeling a lot of sadness, and it's just sitting there in my chest. It feels heavy, like a big blue boulder, and it's cold.* Now take a deep breath into the place in your body where the feeling is concentrated most strongly.

- <u>**Mirror.**</u> Out loud or silently to yourself, say, "I'm feeling sadness (or whatever emotion you're feeling primarily) right now. I won't try to change this feeling; I'm just going to stay with it while it's here." (It's fine to adapt these words to language that feels comfortable to you.) If it feels good, put a hand over your heart as you're speaking. Take another deep breath, then exhale. Feel free to cycle through the steps again as many times as you'd like—or until you start to feel more calm.

Additional option: After moving through all of the steps, ask yourself what color, shape, and sensations you'd like to experience to help you feel as calm and relaxed as possible. Imagine that you have a paintbrush in your hand, and create the picture that feels right to you.

Here's the short version:

- Cancel negative thoughts, taking a big, deep breath.

- Allow your feelings, focusing on which emotion you're feeling *primarily*.

- Link up and listen, connecting with yourself to tune into details about how the emotion feels in your body. Take another deep breath into the place in your body where you're feeling it most strongly.

- Mirror to yourself as the emotion moves through: *Sadness is here, and I'm right here, too.* Breathe again.

Moms we've guided through this process have been amazed at how quickly they calm as they allow their emotions to move through their body rather than resisting them; it often happens within seconds. You may also notice that the next time the emotion comes up with a similar trigger, you don't react as strongly. That's because the disconnect you experienced when feeling alone with this same feeling in the past is being repaired by your own connection now. Just staying present with the emotion allows healing to take place. (To listen to a recorded version of this exercise, please visit our website at www. calmandhappy.com.)

Sometimes a Good Cry
Is Just What the Doctor Ordered

Dealing with big emotions as a mom isn't always convenient. You might get hit with a giant tsunami wave of sadness
while you're at the bank, at the park talking to another mom
you don't know very well, or at a family gathering with your
in-laws, for instance. If you get shanghaied this way, just
breathe and work with CALM internally as best you can (or
one of the other supports from Chapter 3), and if you feel like
you need some privacy, tuck yourself into the bathroom or
a quiet place for a few moments. If your feelings do end up
spilling over in front of others, though, or at a time and place
where you'd rather not have that happen, just let it be. You
won't be the first or only mom to have big emotions, for
goodness' sake, and trying to minimize them will only make
you feel worse. You'll probably feel better after a good cry.

Projecting into the Future

*What if she doesn't take her nap? What if she's waking at night
because she's hungry? What if she never gives up her pacifier, she starts
to choke while the babysitter's feeding her lunch, or we never have enough
money to buy a bigger house?* As a mom, there is an endless list of
things you could potentially worry about, some of them perhaps close
to the realm of possibility and others rather far outside of it. Some
moms spend more time running through this list than doing anything
else—including spending time with the baby!

Maybe you've always been a worrier, or maybe your tendency to worry only kicked in once you became a mom. Or maybe you don't worry all that much, but you'd like to do less of it nonetheless. Whatever the case, the one thing that all worriers have in common, when they are actually doing the worrying, is that they are time traveling into the future. This robs you of precious time with your little one, because it is impossible to worry about the future *and* be completely in the present moment at the same time. The other thing that's happening is that you're allowing fear to pollute your environment, inside and out—and adding to the possibility that whatever you're worried about will actually come to pass.

As we've suggested elsewhere in this book, buying into fear, worry, and negativity is a habit. Allowing fear in leads to negative thinking, which leads to worry and anxiety, which leads to more fear, negative thinking, worry, and anxiety—and the vicious cycle goes round and round. How to stop the madness? Simple: Make a decision to plant yourself firmly in the now, and stay there. Are you there yet—or rather *here*? If you are, good for you! If you're not, or if you were for a nanosecond but then a thought occurred to you that distracted you, welcome to the club. The mind loves to time-travel and take turns chewing on the past or nibbling at the future. Staying present in the now takes discipline, and it also requires giving up the idea that we can actually control the future—or change the past. Consider this scenario:

> Buying into fear, worry, and negativity is a habit.

When Megan's baby, Declan, was born at thirty-three weeks, he was rushed off to the NICU. Declan had difficulty breathing early on and had to be hooked up to ventilators. He's also had some challenges

with his kidney functioning, and it's been a long haul with doctors and
medical check-ups to monitor Declan's progress.

Declan has been home for the last several weeks—slowly getting
healthier but still struggling—and Megan worries constantly that
Declan will have to go back into the hospital.

Now, most people would say that given the unfolding of events here,
Megan has every right to worry, and we wouldn't disagree with that.
But the question is, how does worrying serve her or Declan? Will it
lead to feelings of peace and positivity about the progress he's making,
or stress? Will Declan likely have an easier time getting healthier in a
calm environment, or in a stressful one? Here are some other options
Megan could choose instead:

- Megan could work on her breathing, using the Calming
  Breath exercise whenever she started to feel stressed about
  Declan's health. She could even do this while the baby was
  with her, and who knows? Declan might begin to breathe
  more calmly, too.

- Whenever Megan noticed that Declan seemed happy and
  healthy—such as after a good checkup with the doctor or
  after a good feed—she could create an anchor for herself.
  If a worrisome thought crept in throughout her day, she
  could draw on this anchor as often as she needed to.

- If Megan caught herself starting to worry about Declan, she
  could follow the steps for CALM to connect with herself
  and with him.

- Megan could use Baby OM, enjoying the peaceful feelings
  of the vibration of that sound in her body and in her home
  and sharing those with the baby.

- Megan could do the Heart of Gold meditation to cultivate more peace and calm on a regular basis.

We're not saying you don't have a *right* to worry as a mom; there is plenty that you could potentially worry about as the caretaker of the precious little person under your watch. But the question is whether that worry, and watching worrisome movies about the future in your internal theater, actually benefits you. On occasion, you may find that peering into the future is useful; for instance, packing your diaper bag in the morning and envisioning the playdate you'll be on later that day with another mom and baby, you might remember to include an extra change of clothes. More often than, though, you'll find that worry only causes disconnection, stress, and anxiety, and that by worrying so much about the future you actually miss the gift of the present. Like most moms, you've probably already discovered that the vast majority of what you worry about never actually comes true, so is it worth spending time doing it? Would you want to look back on your baby's childhood and realize you spent a lot of it imagining worst-case scenarios that never arrived?

More often than not, you'll find that by worrying so much about the future you miss the gift of the present.

Don't miss out on time with your little one worrying about the future instead of staying present in the now; it'll go by before you blink. And don't let negative thoughts containing fear and worry convince you that the future is as bleak as they would like you to believe; if you're going to spend time in the future at all, create a positive picture that puts you, your baby, and your family in the best light possible. That will help ensure a bright future indeed.

You Are What You Feel

Which emotions do you label as "good" and "bad"? For the ones that you consider bad, what happens in your body when these feelings start to register? Whatever you are doing—tensing your shoulders or neck, shifting your hips to a tilt, jiggling your left foot—is your particular defense against those feelings. These are also likely the areas that you have the hardest time relaxing. Next time an emotion that you don't like starts to arise, see what happens if you *don't* do the thing you usually do. Can you work with CALM, or another support from Chapter 3, to tolerate the emotion more fully? There is no "right" emotion to feel or state to be in, just the truth of what you're experiencing now.

CHAPTER 8

Stay Calm and Carry On

H opefully, by the time you're reading these words you're feeling more calm and relaxed than you were when you opened this book for the first time. Or maybe you were an already calm mama who's now feeling even more empowered with a few new ideas to try. Either way, the more you get to know what it feels like to be in your center—experiencing whatever you are experiencing, while staying open and nonreactive—the more familiar being there will become.

When you center yourself by working with the steps in CALM, you accomplish three very important things:

1. You naturally feel more relaxed, which allows you to be infinitely more available to mirror and attune to your baby and help her relax, too. Your loving support and caring is what helps your baby learn how to tolerate her own ups and downs.

2. Because you're centered rather than stressed or panicked, you can tap into your mama instincts much more easily, giving you clarity about how best to respond.

3. You learn to tolerate sensations of physical and emotional discomfort, rather than avoiding them; this rewires your brain's neural circuitry, creating a new habit. The more you practice CALM, the more staying present with what you experience will become the norm rather than the exception.

As you've already discovered by now, when you're in sync with your baby, it generally feels great; when you're not, it can feel quite challenging. Even so, because you are the mom, you have the opportunity—and the responsibility—to set the tone and pace of attunement with your baby. Your baby doesn't need you to be an unbreakable rock who never feels challenged or upset herself, but she does need to know that you are bigger than her big feelings and her big experiences. Your baby isn't asking for a mom who's never overwhelmed, but she is asking for reassurance that when a wave of sensory experience or emotion threatens to flood her being, you aren't going to drown along with her. Your baby doesn't need you to be perfect, but she does need you to be present and attuned

> Because you are the mom, you have the opportunity—and the responsibility—to set the tone and pace of attunement with your baby.

to her often enough that she learns how to manage her life experiences, including the uncomfortable ones. When you offer her these gifts, you also help ensure that the legacy she inherits from you is one of strength and resilience that can take her through life's challenges.

You might have noticed that this is actually a book about relationships. It's a book about having a relationship with yourself, first and foremost; when you show up for yourself, you can then show up for your baby, your partner or spouse, and everyone else in a much more authentic way. By no means is it always easy to stand in the truth of whatever it is you're experiencing, especially when what you're experiencing is painful, but the rewards—which include feeling more confident as a mom, more clear about your choices, and able to hear your internal guidance more easily—are well worth the effort.

Staying Calm and Happy

If you find that you've fallen back into more than a little stress from time to time, all is not lost. Just thumb through the pages of this book and see what speaks to you. You may recognize that you've been judging yourself or others, using one of the negative mama mantras; you may realize that you've been pushing down or avoiding some painful feelings; you may become aware that there's a truth you haven't expressed; you may recognize that you've been projecting some of your negativity onto your partner or spouse. Go easy. Be gentle with yourself. Give yourself permission to do it the old way sometimes, whatever that way is, and just pay attention to how that feels. If it doesn't feel good, you can always make a different choice instead.

It's a good idea, too, to check your motivation for using CALM once in a while. If you're a person who tends to like to control things, you might find, if you scratch the surface, that you're actually trying to "get" the baby to calm rather than centering yourself, then connecting with her. Oops. It's not about controlling her experience at all, or even your own; rather, what you're going for is staying *present,* and welcoming calm as a likely byproduct of that choice. Your baby's calm will often follow suit, and if it doesn't, it's not her fault or yours, and you don't have to keep endlessly searching for the smoking gun; you won't always find it. Instead, just stay connected to yourself—and to her—no matter what the experience you're having together brings, and you'll find that "results" matter less and less.

Being a mom is wonderful—and sometimes incredibly hard. And you know what? You can do it. You *are* doing it. When the going gets rough, fasten your seatbelt and get ready to learn something. Make a choice not to buy into fear and limited thinking. Take responsibility for what you see in the mirror of your relationships; get clear about how you feel and what you need, and speak up when necessary. Above all, be kind to yourself. Take the time to appreciate all that you give so generously.

> When the going gets rough, fasten your seatbelt and get ready to learn something.

We salute all moms who navigate their journey through motherhood with determination, dedication, commitment, and love, who do their best despite difficult circumstances and hardship, and who rise to the occasion time and time again, digging deep to discover resources beyond what seems possible.

Thank you for making the world a better place.

Questions and Answers

Q. *I feel so emotional since giving birth, and I'm terrified that if I just let my feelings come, they'll drown me like a giant wave.*

A. Almost every new mom feels this way, especially during the first few months. But here's the thing: the alternative to feeling your feelings is to *not* feel them—shutting them down or distracting yourself—and if you've had any experience with doing those things, you've probably discovered just how stressed and anxious that can make you feel. It's actually the practice of avoiding your feelings that can cause a giant flood: when your feelings are backed up for long stretches of time, the dam eventually bursts and they spill over everywhere. Allowing your emotions to arise and staying present with them is what will help you feel more balanced on an ongoing basis.

Q. *What if I start crying when I'm with my baby? Won't that be upsetting for her—and cause her to cry, too?*

A. If you cry in front of her and beat yourself up for it, she will definitely pick up on that. But feelings are only "negative" when we believe we shouldn't have them. When you have feelings as you're with the baby and take responsibility for them by staying present rather than avoiding them or reacting, she learns that it's okay to have emotions, too, and to express them. You can say to her, "Mommy's feeling sad right now, honey; this isn't about you. I'm taking care of myself by letting my tears come, because it's okay to cry when you're sad." When you give yourself permission to feel your feelings, rather than shutting them down because you think you should "be strong" for her as the mom, you help them surface, then release; when they aren't stopped, feelings come and go in a very fluid way. If you're feeling a particularly strong wave of sadness or frustration and there's another adult with you to watch the baby, you can excuse yourself to a different room for a few minutes if you need some private time to get your bearings.

Q: *My baby is colicky and cries constantly. It's so hard not to feel stressed when there's never a break.*

A: Having a baby who cries a lot or is colicky, a child with a medical issue, or other stressors going on in your family, such as financial issues or a move, can feel especially challenging. Remember, the supports in this book are not designed to ensure that you always feel perfectly calm but rather are to help you be honest about what you're experiencing, and be *present* with it. Giving yourself permission to feel stressed and irritated, and acknowledging those feelings in your body, may ironically help you feel calmer and more at peace—and may even affect your baby's mood in a positive way, too. Be sure to take breaks often, whether taking turns being "on duty" with the baby's other parent or asking another adult to take over for a while.

Q: *I have a hard time not feeling guilty whenever I'm having negative thoughts or emotions. I just keep thinking about all that negativity passing through the invisible umbilical and harming my baby. Help!*

A: That's the catch-22: it's good to know that your energy affects the baby, but knowing that, you can have "stage fright" as you allow yourself to be honest about the internal experience you're having as a mom. *Every* mom has negative thoughts and emotions at times, and stress. Remember, it's not *that* you feel these things that affect the baby but what you do with them; acknowledging them is the key to letting them go.

Q: *Have I already done damage by allowing my negative thoughts and feelings to affect my baby?*

A: Thinking that way sounds a lot like *I'm doing it wrong* and is a surefire recipe for nothing but stress. The quality of your attachment to your baby is most strongly influenced by how you are managing your mood and emotional state right *now*. What's more, the baby's brain is incredibly resilient at this young age; as you begin to change old habits of stress and negativity, she will benefit greatly from those choices.

Q: *Sometimes being a mom is really hard, and I don't have the strength to go through CALM or stay present with what I'm feeling. When I'm stressed, sometimes I just want to eat chocolate and read a stupid magazine! What happens to the baby if I make this choice?*

A: She gets to have some downtime on her play mat while Mommy recharges! As long as you are proactively monitoring your stress *most* of the time, you're doing a great job of providing a healthy environment for your baby to grow up in. Having that strong foundation helps you during times when you get overwhelmed.

Q: *Recently my baby was diagnosed with reflux. The doctor said it might be related to all the dairy I've been eating, since I'm nursing. How can I not blame myself for her condition?*

A: We're willing to bet that you did not wake up one day and say to yourself, *I know what I'll do—I'll eat lots of dairy so the baby's tummy becomes upset.* Instead, you didn't know that eating those foods would irritate her. In other words, you didn't know what you didn't know, and the decisions you were making as a mom were with your best intentions. As a mom, you are constantly in new, uncharted waters, and you're doing the best you can with the information you have; now that you have new information, you can experiment with changing your diet if you wish. There's a big difference between learning from experience and *blaming* yourself for doing something "wrong." Be easy with yourself!

Q: *I was raised by a mother who criticized me a lot, so that became my "programming." I've been criticizing myself since childhood; how can I change such an old habit?*

A: One breath at a time. Now that you're aware that that's your pattern, you can make a conscious choice *not* to hang onto negative thoughts as they come up but to cancel them, breathe, and let them go instead. This probably won't happen overnight; it will take some practice, and while you're on your way you'll likely still catch yourself buying into negative self-talk at times. That's okay; learning new skills takes patience. Whenever you decide not to hang onto negative thoughts but to let them go instead, you create new neural pathways; in time, that choice will become your new habit.

Q: *I feel like a pretty calm mom, but my baby tends to fuss quite a bit. How can this be?*

A: While babies are picking up on your energy all the time, there are other factors influencing a baby's mood, too; these include her individual disposition, the emotions and behaviors of others in the baby's orbit, and how well a baby sleeps and feeds, as well as medical issues. We've met some calm mamas whose babies cry a lot and some stressed-out moms whose babies seem amazingly calm and happy. But your habits of managing stress, or succumbing to it, are what will shape your baby's own tendencies as she grows. If your baby is fussy and you routinely stay present with her through her difficult experiences, you are absolutely teaching her how to manage her ups and downs. Modeling these skills, and maintaining a loving connection with her no matter what, will only benefit her as she grows; your fussy newborn may become a rather calm baby in time!

Q: *I get it about my energy affecting the baby, but my husband doesn't. He tends to run a lot of anxiety and stress, and the baby is often fussy around him. When I try to explain why this is happening, he just gets defensive. What do I do?*

A: What may be happening is that your husband feels bad that he is somehow harming your baby, and that's too much for him to bear. Try coming at the subject from a different angle: On those occasions when he is calmer and more settled, help him connect the dots. "Wow, honey, it's so amazing—we're sitting here so calmly, and look how calm the baby is. She hasn't fussed all morning!" (Okay, that's a little obvious, but you get the idea.) Also, if you're home with the baby and your husband is working out of the home, he may not have as much practice with reading the baby's needs as you do—and therefore may not feel as confident about attending to her. Avoid the temptation to "rescue" the baby from his arms whenever she seems upset; instead, be supportive and give him time to find his way.

Q: *My mom is really loud and enthusiastic with the baby, and some-times the baby starts to cry when we visit. How can I protect her?*

A. Try being honest, respectful, and direct: "You know, Mom, I've noticed that when someone comes at the baby with lots of enthusiasm, she cries. Her nervous system isn't all that developed yet, and it's easy to forget how much bigger we are than she is. Maybe you can tone it down a bit so she can warm up more gradually." The other thing is, unless the baby is absolutely miserable in Grandma's company, you don't necessarily have to do anything to protect her; it's okay to allow her to have upset feelings, then recover—with your help, but only if she needs it. Every time she feels big feelings and recovers, she learns something. Do watch your projections onto your mom along the lines of *You're doing it wrong*—your expectation of what will happen could actually be adding more stress into the mix!

Q. *My caregiver spends a lot of time with my baby, and I want her to use the ideas in this book, but I don't know if she will. Will the baby be affected by her energy since she spends so much time in her company?*

A. While it's true that the baby will pick up on the energy of anyone she's with, you and her other parent have the most influence on her, by far. That being said, it's a good idea to choose a caregiver who's not just qualified on paper but who feels like someone *you* would want to spend time with; if you observe her and the baby together and feel positive about their interaction, that's a good indication that she's a good fit for your family. If you don't, or if your own interactions with your caregiver often feel stressful, you may want to consider hiring someone else.

Appendix A:
Calm and **Happy**
Feeding and Sleep

Calm Sleep

To some of the little bright lights coming onto the planet these days, sleep seems to be something for people who have nothing better to do with their time, which certainly doesn't include them. Your baby may wake up in the morning well before the birds, fight naps with incredible force, and put sleep somewhere on the priority list just after "let mom cut my nails." And yet, despite her lack of shut-eye, your baby may seem bright as a button pretty much around the clock; the combination of her lack of sleep and high energy can seem to defy all logic.

Years ago, we would have said that a baby older than four months and weighing more than fourteen pounds who was not getting the right quality and the right amount of sleep was suffering from poor "sleep nutrition." Today, though, some babies seem to function remarkably well on surprisingly little shut-eye, and trying to force them to sleep more than their bodies seem to need naturally can be quite an uphill battle. Even if your child seems strangely buoyant after partying like a rock star all night long, though, *you* may feel like you're barely keeping up.

What you may also have found is that, despite your best efforts, your baby's erratic sleep patterns don't begin to match the schedules that some parenting books—including the one Jennifer coauthored, *The Sleepeasy Solution*—so helpfully suggest. What's more, even after following your chosen sleep book's instructions to the letter, your baby may still wake at night, take short naps, or wake early in the morning long before you're ready to rise and shine. The cherry on top? When your little one finally seems to fall into a rhythm, she may suddenly fall out of it again, and there may not always be a clear reason why (no new tooth, no illness to explain the change). With all of this unpredictability, you may sometimes wonder whether you've been cursed by the sleep gods!

Whether your baby clearly shows signs of being overtired or whether she's thriving despite her lack of sleep, the ideas in this section can help both you and your baby to get more peaceful sleep. They are designed to work in conjunction with whatever other methods you feel comfortable using to help improve your baby's sleep skills and will nicely complement any plan that you're following. They can also significantly diminish your potential upset feelings about this subject, and your little one's as well, as you gently guide her toward better sleep. It's not necessary that you follow all of the ideas to see improvement; try whatever resonates and skip whatever doesn't.

How Stress Can Affect Your Baby's Sleep

Since one theme of this book is the effect of mom's mood and energy on her baby, you may be wondering whether your mood and emotions have an effect on your baby's sleep, too. Indeed they do.[19] If your baby has trouble sleeping, would you believe us if we told you that if you did *nothing else* but manage your energy, plus believe wholeheartedly that she could sleep better, that she would? That might sound hard to imagine, but we've absolutely seen a correlation between mom and dad's calm, or stress, and their little one's patterns of sleep or wakefulness. Generally speaking, relaxed parents tend to have babies who sleep better than stressed parents do. Please know that we aren't *blaming* you for your baby's poor sleep if you're experiencing some stress in this area; we're simply suggesting that choosing to feel less stressed about it may help improve things a bit.

Sleep can be an emotionally charged subject for many moms, because so much of your baby's well-being seems to depend on it. Here are some other possible reasons why:

- One or more of the people in your orbit—your mother, your mother-in-law, your husband, your best friend, your pediatrician—says that your baby "should" be sleeping through the night. That's a myth. Many babies *can* sleep long stretches beginning at four months and fourteen pounds, but if you are getting up a couple of times a night to feed and both you and the baby go back to sleep quickly, you do not necessarily have a sleep problem.* If your baby shows signs

---

* Please don't begin a formal sleep-learning program with your baby until she is at least four months old (adjusting for any prematurity) and weighs at least fourteen pounds, to allow for cognitive and physical development that will best support her learning. Some babies with sensitive nervous systems, especially those who were born prematurely or have medical issues, are better off waiting until closer to six months to begin learning.

of chronic sleep deprivation, though, or either you or your partner or spouse is exhausted, then you may want to take steps to improve things.

- Unless you're cosleeping, sleep is a separation. If you or the baby experienced medical issues or trauma during pregnancy or delivery, separating from your baby for sleep can trigger painful memories. (We are not for or against cosleeping, by the way; either choice works well for a family as long as each family member is aligned with that choice.)

- If you either felt neglected as a child or had a parent who rarely left your side, separating for sleep may feel difficult for you, as you may believe on some level that you are abandoning your child.

- The idea of allowing your baby to fuss for a few minutes as she settles herself to sleep may feel challenging for you for a variety of reasons.

- If your baby chronically fights sleep, you may worry that she's not getting enough rest and that her lack of sleep is adversely affecting her health and development.

- If your baby needs lots of help settling and/or wakes often, you may feel resentful because it seems like you're never off duty as a mom.

Whether you're aware of it or not, your baby's sleep may be bringing up all kinds of emotions—and stress—for you, and possibly for your husband or partner, too. Working with CALM, or any of the supports from Chapter 3 (especially the breathing exercises), can help.

Calm Mama, Sleepy Baby

If your baby is older than four months and weighs at least fourteen pounds, seems well rested and happy upon waking, and makes it easily to the next sleep period without lots of emotional or behavioral ups and downs, then she is most likely getting the right amount of sleep for her regardless of what the books or experts say, and you don't need to do anything differently. (For babies under four months, there are no "bad habits" or schedules to adhere to; feel free to help your baby to sleep however necessary.) On the other hand, some babies unfortunately do have a hard time settling, wake in distress, and truly don't seem rested on the sleep they're getting. Whatever the case for your little one, these suggestions can help you both get better shut-eye.

- If your baby historically has not been a great sleeper, you are likely (and understandably) running a lot of anxiety and worry each time you put her down; if so, she may be picking up on that. No matter how challenging your baby's sleep has been up until this moment, at least 20 minutes before putting your baby down for sleep, begin visualizing a smooth, easy, peaceful flow to your wind-down. See the baby settling into sleep peacefully and sleeping well throughout the night or her nap. Your ability to hold this vision counts for a lot! If you believe she can sleep well, it's much more likely that she will.

- Note that some babies wake in the night and do not cry or seem distressed. If your child is doing this, *and she seems rested and happy in the morning,* let her be! Going to her when she's not asking for help can inadvertently contribute to the wakeups.

- At least 15 minutes before putting your baby down to sleep, use your anchor to help you calm and relax. If you'd like, use your baby's anchor, too.

- At least 10 minutes before putting your baby down to sleep, begin breathing deeply. You can also use the Calming Breath to help you relax even further. Continue to breathe deeply throughout your wind-down routine.

- Throughout your wind-down routine, cycle through the steps for CALM, cancelling negative thoughts, allowing your feelings, linking up and listening, and mirroring with the baby. This will help both of you stay as relaxed and connected as possible.

- In a calm, loving, and direct way, have a conversation with the baby in which you explain any changes that you'll be making with her sleep, such as putting her down more wakeful. Because of the invisible umbilical that connects you both, your baby understands far more of what you say than you may imagine! She may not understand every word just yet, but she will certainly understand the tone in your voice and the energy behind what you're saying.

- Whatever method you decide to use to help your baby learn how to sleep, at whatever point she fusses, continue to take deep breaths and cycle through the steps for CALM. For linking up and listening and mirroring, you can do these steps even if the baby isn't in the same room with you; because of the invisible umbilical, she can feel you communicating with her—and sending her love—even if you're not in the same space. You can also work with Using CALM for Managing Emotions in Chapter 7 to help you deal with strong feelings that may come up while she's learning.

- As the baby is learning, you can work with the Heart of Gold meditation, envisioning that you are sharing your calm, peaceful energy with the baby and enveloping her in calm, too. You can use this exercise whether you're in the same room together or in separate rooms for a few minutes at a time while she learns.

- As your baby begins to learn how to be a better sleeper, over the following few days you can work with the Tuning in Within exercise to access clear guidance about any adjustments that might help your baby sleep as well as possible. Don't be afraid to experiment!

- Remember to manage your expectations about the amount of sleep your little bright light needs. Despite your best efforts, she may wake at 5:30 in the morning bright eyed and bushy tailed, and she may never nap longer than 45 minutes. If she genuinely seems rested when she wakes from any sleep period and easily makes it until the next one, she's getting the right amount of sleep for her—regardless of what the experts say.

Tuning In Within for Guidance on Your Baby's Sleep

If you've been using a tried-and-true sleep method to help your baby sleep and you aren't seeing progress, or if you'd simply like to consult your own guidance about this subject, you can try working with this exercise (from Chapter 3) to see what you may be able to discover about your baby's particular sleep patterns and needs.

- Sitting comfortably, take three deep breaths. Close your eyes on the third exhale breath.

- Frame your request for guidance as a clear question: for example, *How can I help the baby sleep better at night?*

- Now tune in and listen; stay open to whatever comes. You might hear words, you might get an idea, you might see a picture, you might get a feeling or just a sense of knowing— whatever kind of guidance comes is perfect for you. You don't have to analyze or evaluate the guidance you get in this step; just let the ideas come. Here are some examples of what you might get:

  - *She might be overtired. She seems to get fussy about a half hour before we're putting her down, then gets a second wind. Maybe we should adjust bedtime earlier.*

  - *She has a really hard time getting out of the bath and transitioning into PJs. Maybe it would be easier to put her PJs on in the bathroom, where it's warmer, rather than bringing her to the room.*

  - *Daddy sometimes tries to "cheer her up" by tickling her or making funny sounds, and he's coming from a place of love, but she might be getting overstimulated if she's tired. Maybe he can sing to her instead.*

If you're not used to tuning in to your internal guidance this way, it may seem hard to imagine at first that you'll actually get much valuable information. Stay open and give yourself time to practice; you might be surprised by what you discover!

An Unbreakable Bond

Although your physical bodies may not always be in the same place at the same time, you and the baby are never actually separate; instead, you are *always* connected in your hearts. This is a powerful truth that you can start teaching the baby even now, at this very young age. Remembering your connection via the invisible umbilical will serve both you and the baby—and your relationship—very well as she continues to develop and grow.

Calm Feeding

Just as with sleep, the energy you're holding—whether tense or calm—can have a clear effect on your baby's ability to feed well, whether you're feeding her milk or solids. Stressed-out mamas tend to have babies who don't feed as well, and long-term stress can affect a nursing mom's milk supply. Here are some tips to help your feeding times with the baby flow as smoothly as possible.

- Ten to twenty minutes before feeding time, visualize your feeding session with the baby going very smoothly: see her latching on or taking the bottle easily, feeding calmly, and the two of you enjoying the closeness of your skin-to-skin contact. Even if things have been challenging up till now, get into the feeling place of what it would be like to have more peaceful feedings: *Wow, I can't believe how well that went! The baby fed really well. Seems like we've really turned a corner.* Imagine sharing this good news with your husband, your mom, and your pediatrician.

- Ten to 15 minutes before you're ready to feed the baby, use your anchor to help you calm and relax. Just as with sleep, you can use your baby's anchor, too.

- Alternatively, do the Heart of Gold Meditation or Baby OM exercise to get in sync with your baby.

- At least 10 minutes before beginning to feed your baby, begin breathing deeply. You can also use the Calming Breath exercise to help you relax even further. Continue to breathe deeply throughout your feeding session.

- If feeding has been challenging, in a calm, loving and direct way, talk to the baby to connect with her before your feeding session begins. Focus on the tone in your voice and the energy behind what you're saying. For instance, try telling her that whether she feeds steadily or needs to take some breaks, it's okay to take her time. Giving the baby permission to feed in the way she needs to can help take the pressure off of any "performance" aspect of the feeding process for you both.

- As you begin to feed, cycle through the steps for CALM, cancelling negative thoughts (i.e., that it might not go well), allowing your feelings (including any anxiety—breathe into it), linking up and listening (continuing to tune in to the baby while she feeds or making any necessary adjustments in your or her position, for instance), and mirroring with the baby while she feeds (whether talking to her or simply using your eye contact or touch). Continue to breathe deeply as you cycle through the steps.

- While you're feeding the baby, hold the intention that you are offering her lots of love and positivity along with your milk.

- When your feeding session feels relaxed and peaceful, you can reinforce your feelings of calm and confidence by using your anchor, and possibly hers as well.

Appendix B:
Color and Music

Color

The colors in our environment can have a profound effect on our mood and energy, and if your little bright light is in motion from the minute she wakes up in the morning till the end of her day, you'll want to consider how the colors in her environment—including walls, carpets, and furniture—may be affecting her.

All of us, even babies, have natural different responses to certain colors; because of our individual wiring, we're more drawn to certain colors and not as drawn to others. The colors that we're naturally drawn to can tell us something about our personalities; we can then use color to balance our energy and emotions. This is true for babies and adults alike.

Here's an experiment you can try: Get some fabric swatches of various colors at your local fabric shop (making sure that they're large enough not to be a hazard to the baby) and scatter them around the room where your baby is playing. Then watch and see which colors she tends to be attracted to the most; it may take a few days to see which colors she seems to be drawn to repeatedly. What she gravitates toward can give you an indication as to her personality—both balances and imbalances—and provide you with information that will help you decide what colors to use in her bedroom, in the area where she plays, and in her general environment.

Here are some examples of what different colors may indicate:

Green: support, balance, harmony, love, social tendencies, an affinity for nature, acceptance, growth, money, healing

Yellow: fun, humor, laughter, logic, creativity, nurturance, personal power

Red: high energy, vitality, grounding, stability yet also spontaneity

Violet: intuition, imagination, artistic balance

Light turquoise blue: calm, peace, depth, devotion, confidence restfulness

Pink: romance, compassion, friendship, sensitivity

White: clear mindedness, freshness, goodness, simplicity, purity

Cream: new beginnings, constant change

Black: an inquisitive mind that wants to break the mysteries of life

Orange: warmth, liveliness, being energetic, outgoing and free spirited

If you're reading this book as a mama-to-be, rather than creating your baby's nursery now with the colors you like, you can wait till the baby arrives, tune in, and see what colors you feel would help her thrive. If your little one is already here, you may want to consider whether the colors in her environment are the ideal ones for her. For example, a child who enjoys constant change may feel restless in a nursery where cream is the dominant color, and a highly energetic child may feel even more stimulated in a room with reds and oranges but calmer where shades of blue are used.

Music

Remember when we talked about the sound *om* in Chapter 3? *Om* is the vibration of sound that the universe makes, and a field of scientific study called quantum mechanics tells us that everything in the universe is indeed vibrating at different speeds. All of those different vibrations make up the notes in our musical scales.

You know that toy piano or xylophone in your baby's toy box? Next time your baby is playing with it, do an experiment. Take turns striking each of the notes, and see how your baby responds. You'll likely find that certain notes seem to get her attention more—perhaps exciting her, perhaps helping her relax into calm. Play the notes repeatedly, so you can accurately gauge her response to them. When you find the notes that help her calm, you can play those—or hum them—in times when she's fussing to help her relax. If you have other, adult-size instruments in the house, feel free to experiment with these as well.

Note that your baby's response to different musical notes may change over time, as she grows and develops—so check in periodically to see how her response has changed.

Appendix C:
Caring Papa
Happy Mama

A dad who is a new parent has his own unique journey into parenthood. Just as happens with moms, a dad's heart cracks open with the baby's arrival, and with that comes all kinds of strong emotions—as well as a dramatically different perspective on what matters in life.

From a dad's point of view, the connection a mom has with the new baby can feel a bit mysterious; moms carry the baby for forty weeks, give birth to her, and nurse—all experiences that a dad will never have and can't fully understand. But hopefully it goes without saying that a dad's connection to his child is strong and special in its own right, and whether you're the kind of dad who changes diapers and takes turns rocking the baby to sleep or whether you spend time with her in other ways, you are nurturing your relationship with your child in your own way. At the same time, just as is true for moms, your baby is paying close attention to your thoughts, emotions, and behavior, so it's a good idea to be mindful about the energy you're bringing to your connection. (We'll be addressing the nuances of the papa-baby relationship in an upcoming book especially for you.)

Since this is a book for moms, and since the quality of the parents' relationship influences both a mom's and baby's well-being so strongly, we thought we would share some of the observations we've made over the years about what helps moms feel as connected to dads as possible in the early weeks and months of welcoming a new baby. Since Derek is a dad (and granddad) himself, many of these observations are offered from firsthand experience. There's no magic formula that creates a happy relationship, but attuning to your wife's needs as she adjusts to being a new mom can go a long way toward shoring up your connection—and the stronger that connection is, the more both of you, and your baby, will thrive.

- Because moms are so intricately involved in the physical caretaking of the baby, your contributions to your wife's well-being cannot be underestimated. There are two primary paths you can choose: to take turns helping to take care of the baby, or to go out of your way to help your wife feel as comfortable and supported as possible. If you don't know what would help her feel comfortable and supported, ask!

- In the first few weeks and months especially, don't take it personally if you'd like to be more involved with the baby than your wife prefers, or conversely if she chastises you for not being more involved than you are. You're both finding your way as new parents and adjusting to the changes in your relationship as well—not to mention figuring out how to accommodate the needs of a tiny new person. Keep the lines of communication open; it may take some time for you to find the balance that feels right to you both.

- If your wife feels strongly about handling a certain aspect of taking care of the baby, such as how and where she sleeps, follow her lead. There may be other areas of parenting that you feel strongly about, so save your energy for speaking up about those instead.

- Because a mom's body undergoes so many changes during pregnancy and in the weeks and months following birth, she doesn't always feel physically attractive. (You know that she is, of course, but moms can be very hard on themselves in this department.) Remind her often how beautiful she is.

- The only exception to the previous point is that you should *not* offer compliments as a way to open the door to intimacy. Don't push for sex too often or too soon after the new baby arrives. The physicality of taking care of a baby is indescribably exhausting for a mom, so it can feel like a pretty major gear-shift for her to go from holding and nursing the baby to connecting physically with you. If you're brand-new parents, other kinds of physical closeness—snuggling while you watch a movie, for instance—can be a good interim way to connect until sex feels right to you both.

- If your wife stays home with the baby and you work out of the home, don't assume that she has the easier job. Keeping up with the demands of a baby all day long can be incredibly stressful, even if your wife loves being a mom.

- When you come home at the end of the day, whether your wife works out of the home or works at home as a mom, greet her warmly before spending time with your child. It feels good to kick off your evening together this way, and there's an added bonus: when children see mom and dad connecting warmly, they feel happy and safe.

- If you're the kind of person who needs ten minutes after walking in the door to shift gears from work to family time, communicate this to your wife so she doesn't have different expectations about what should happen as soon as you come home. If you both work out of the home, take turns by giving each other a few minutes of downtime at the end of the day.

Here is some additional feedback for dads from some of the moms we've worked with:

- We moms really need your help! You may not have a breast and you may have to work during the day, but we still need you to walk, rock, watch, and hold the baby without grumbling. If you don't get this practice early on, when the baby is older you won't be able to console her easily. If your wife is the only one who can comfort the baby, there will be very little time left for you!

- Be proactive. In the beginning especially, we may be too preoccupied to think about what's for dinner. Go to the market or take the lead in ordering takeout. Offer to give the baby a bath, or at least get the diaper, wipes, and PJs ready. When it feels like we're in it together as parents, it feels really good.

- Let us know you care. We need some spoiling! The smallest thing, like bringing us a glass of water or an extra pillow while we're nursing, can make such a difference. Give me a foot massage, and you're my hero.

- "What can I do for you?" goes a very long way.

- Just be a good listener and don't try to "fix it." When we talk about how hard it is being a mom, we're just sharing and usually not looking for a solution. Listening to us *is* doing something, even if it doesn't feel that way to you.

Resources

American Academy of Pediatrics, www.aap.org

Calm Mama, Happy Baby, www.calmandhappy.com

Healthy Child, Healthy World, www.Healthychild.org

KellyMom.com, www.kellymom.com

La Leche League International, www.lalecheleague.org

MomAssembly.com, www.momassembly.com

National Organization of Mothers of Twins Clubs (NOMOTC), www.nomotc.com

The Period of Purple Crying, www.purplecrying.info

Positively Positive, www.positivelypositive.com

Postpartum Support International, www.postpartum.net

SIDS Alliance, www.sidsalliance.com

Sleepy Planet, www.sleepyplanet.com

Zero to Three, www.zerotothree.org

Books

10 Mindful Minutes: Giving Our Children—and Ourselves—the Social and Emotional Skills to Reduce Stress and Anxiety *by Goldie Hawn*

A clear explanation of how our thoughts, emotions, and actions are interconnected, as well as simple ways to cultivate mindfulness.

Becoming Attached: First Relationships and How They Shape Our Capacity to Love *by Robert Karen*

Insightful discussion about how the parent-child relationship helps to shape who we are.

The Biology of Belief *by Bruce Lipton*

Scientific discoveries about the interaction between the mind and the body, and how our cells receive information from our thoughts.

Brain Rules for Baby *by John Medina*

The author, a molecular biologist and dad, explores what the latest science shows about how a baby's brain works.

Good Nights: The Happy Parents' Guide to the Family Bed
by Jay Gordon

Guidance from a well-known pediatrician on how to share a family bed safely—and keep the spark in your marriage.

Happiness *by Derek O'Neill*

How to stop chasing happiness, which is fleeting, and instead find the balance in life's ups and downs that leads to long-term joy. Part of the "Get a Grip" series; other titles include *Confidence, Depression,* and *Relationships.*

My Stroke of Insight *by Jill Bolte Taylor*

Fascinating story of a neuroscientist who had a stroke and, as a recovering patient, experienced an extremely high level of sensory perception—similar to what a child experiences.

Parenting from the Inside Out *by Dan Siegel and Mary Hartzell*

Wonderful exploration, grounded in neuroscience, of how a parent's past informs their present as they interact with their child.

The Sleepeasy Solution: The Exhausted Parent's Guide to Getting Your Child to Sleep *by Jennifer Waldburger and Jill Spivack*

Step-by-step guidance on how to help your baby sleep through the night and take great naps. DVD available as well.

The Whole-Brain Child *by Dan Siegel and Tina Payne Bryson*

Gives parents tools for understanding their child's brain and how to apply this knowledge to create healthy parent-child relationships and interactions.

Your One-Year-Old *by Lousie Bates Ames, PhD*

This condensed book guides you through the developmental issues that parents face during the first year. Series includes books for other ages as well.

Your Self-Confident Baby *by Magda Gerber and Allison Johnson*

Fascinating information about nurturing a child's natural instincts.

Notes

Chapter 1

[1] Peter A. Wyman, Jane Moynihan et al., "Association of Family Stress with Natural Killer Cell Activity and the Frequency of Illnesses in Children," *JAMA Pediatrics,* March 2007.

[2] This study showed differential methylation in adolescents where there had been reports of parental high stress during their child's infancy and early childhood. M. J. Essex, W. T. Boyce et al., "Epigenetic Vestiges of Early Developmental Adversity: Childhood Stress Exposure and DNA Methylation in Adolescence," *Child Development*, September 2011.

[3] American Psychological Association, "Stress in America," Washington, DC, November 2010.

[4] J. S. Middlebrooks and N. C. Audage, "The Effects of Childhood Stress on Health Across the Lifespan," Centers for Disease Control and Prevention, National Center for Injury Prevention and Control, Atlanta, GA, 2008.

Chapter 2

[5] Christine Moon, Hugo Lagercratnz, and Patricia K. Kuhl, "Language Experienced in Utero Affects Language Perception after Birth," *Acta Paediatrica*, February 2013.

Janet L. Hopson, "Fetal Psychology," *Psychology Today*, October 1998.

Kazuyuki Shinorhara, "Fetal Response to Induced Maternal Emotions," *The Journal of Physiological Sciences,* May 2010: vol. 60, issue 3, pp. 213–220.

Vivette Glover and Thomas O'Connor, "Effects of Antenatal Stress and Anxiety," *British Journal of Psychiatry* 2002, pp. 389–91.

[6] According to researcher Dan Siegel, "The mirror neuron system is thought to be an essential aspect of the neural basis for empathy. By perceiving the expressions of another individual, the brain is able to create within its own body an internal state that is thought to 'resonate' with that of the other person." D. J. Siegel, "An Interpersonal Neurobiology Approach to Psychotherapy: How Awareness, Mirror Neurons and Neural Plasticity Contribute to the Development of Well-Being," *Psychiatric Annals* 36, no. 4, 2006.

J. E. Swain et al., "Brain Basis of Early Parent-Child Interactions: Psychology, Physiology, and In Vivo Functional Neuroimaging Studies," *Journal of Child Psychology and Psychiatry and Allied Disciplines* 48, March-April 2007.

Gerald J. Haeffel and Jennifer L. Harnes, "Cognitive Vulnerability to Depression Can Be Contagious," *Clinical Psychological Science,* April 16, 2013.

Sigal G. Barsade, "The Ripple Effect: Emotional Contagion and Its Influence on Group Behavior," *Administrative Science Quarterly,* vol. 47, no. 4, December 2002.

[7] Jill Bolte Taylor, *My Stroke of Insight: A Brain Scientist's Personal Journey.* Plume, 2009.

[8] Daniel Goleman, drawing from the work of Joseph E. LeDoux, writes about this phenomenon, which he calls an "amygdala hijack," in his book *Emotional Intelligence: Why It Can Matter More Than IQ.* Bantam, 1996.

[9] Daniel J. Siegel and Mary Payne Bryson, *The Whole-Brain Child: 12 Revolutionary Strategies to Nurture Your Child's Developing Mind, Survive Everyday Parenting Struggles, and Help Your Family Thrive.* Random House, 2011.

Chapter 3

[10] This term was coined by psychiatrist and researcher Dan Siegel, who has presented his groundbreaking work about empathy and the brain in many books and publications, including *The Developing Mind: How Relationships and the Brain Interact to Shape Who We Are* (Guilford Press, 2012) and *Parenting from the Inside Out,* which he coauthored with Mary Hartzell (Tarcher, 2004).

[11] Silvan S. Tomkins, in *Affect, Imagery, Consciousness, Vol. 2: The Negative Affects.* Springer, 1963.

Allan N. Shore, *Affect Dysregulation and Disorders of the Self.* W. W. Norton, 2003.

[12] V. S. Ramachandran, "The Neurology of Self-Awareness," *Edge* website, 2007, essay available at http://www.edge.org/3rd_culture/ramachandran07/ramachandran07_index.html.

[13] D. W. Winnicott, "The Theory of the Parent-Infant Relationship," *International Journal of Psycho-Analysis* 41, 1960.

[14] David M. Levy, Jacob O. Wobbrock, Alfred W. Kaszniak, and Marilyn Ostregren, "The Effects of Mindfulness Meditation Training on Multitasking in a High-Stress Information Environment," *Proceedings of Graphics Interface,* May 2012.

Adam Burke, "Comparing Individual Preferences for Four Meditation Techniques: Zen, Vipassana (Mindfulness), Qigong, and Mantra," *Explore: The Journal of Science and Healing,* vol. 8, issue 4, July 2012.

Chapter 5
[15] Harvey Karp. *The Happiest Baby on the Block.* Bantam, 2003.

Chapter 6
[16] Alice A. Graham, Philip A. Fischer, and Jennifer H. Pfeifer, "What Sleeping Babies Hear: A Functional MRI Study of Interparental Conflict and Infants' Emotion Processing," *Psychological Science,* July 2012.

Margaret Tresch Owen and Martha J. Cox, "Marital Conflict and the Development of Infant-Parent Attachment Relationships," *Journal of Family Psychology,* vol. 11(2), June 1997.

[17] John Gottman, *The 7 Principles for Making Marriage Work.* Three Rivers Press, 2000.

Chapter 7
[18] Deepak Chopra, *Quantum Healing: Exploring the Frontiers of Mind/Body Medicine.* Bantam, 1990.

Bruce Lipton, *The Biology of Belief: Unleashing the Power of Consciousness, Matter and Miracles.* Hay House, 2008.

Lissa Rankin, *Mind Over Medicine: Scientific Proof That You Can Heal Yourself.* Hay House, 2013.

Appendix
[19] Roseanne Armitage, Heather Flynn, Robert Hoffman, Delia Vazquez, Juan Lopez, and Sheila Marcus, "Early Developmental Changes in Sleep in Infants: The Impact of Maternal Depression," *SLEEP,* May 2009.

Acknowledgments

Derek would like to thank:

My two children, Gavin and Orla, for their endless support, love, and insightfulness.

My two grandchildren, Alexa and Blake.

My late wife, Linda, who was and continues to be my greatest inspiration.

My mum, dad, sisters, and brothers.

All who have changed their lives for the better by applying what I teach in their own lives.

All the children in the world who suffer and have suffered, for giving me an opportunity to exercise compassion in action.

Last but not least, all at SQ Worldwide and SQ Foundation for their support through the path of knowledge.

Jennifer would like to thank:

My family, Anne, Richard, Stefanie, and Erica, for their continued love and support, and for always believing in me.

Derek O'Neill, for inspiring me.

Linda O'Neill, who is always in my heart.

Jill Spivack, whose friendship and partnership make me a better person, and Gary, for always cheering us on.

Jake and Emma Spivack, for being who you are.

Louise Waldburger, Connie Tregenza, Lena Young, Margaret Via, Roslyn Luke, Sharon Kleitsch, Lois Thompson, Liora Elghanayan,

Donna Friedman, Carol Patton, Susan Robertson, and all the grand-mothers who paved the way.

All of the moms, babies, and children—and dads, too—I have had the honor and privilege of knowing and working with. You have taught me so much about love, courage, and sacrifice, and I am so grateful for the gift of sharing your journey.

Derek and Jennifer would like to thank:

Maren Kannow, Zelana Montminy, Suzanne Selmo, Krista Santino, Ian Hoge, Shawn Gardner, Anthony Smokovich, Jenna Lecce, Katherine Hamer, Sherri Greene, Anjalee Galion and Allison Mitchell, for your editorial eyes and contributions to this book.

Allison Janse, Kim Weiss, Larissa Henoch, Lawna Oldfield, and everyone at HCI for your enthusiasm for this project.

Bill Abrams, Charissa Barton, and Jonathan Keenan, for all of your wonderful support.

Index

About the Authors

For more than fifteen years, **Derek O'Neill** has been transforming the lives of thousands of people around the world for the better. An internationally acclaimed psychotherapist, motivational speaker, author, martial arts sensei, and humanitarian, Derek inspires and uplifts people from all walks of life through his books, workshops, consultations, speaking engagements, media appearances, and tireless humanitarian work.

Drawing on thirty years of training in martial arts, which earned him the level of Master Black Belt, and incorporating his extraordinary intuitive abilities and expertise as a psychotherapist, Derek has pioneered a new psychology, transformational therapy. His signature "Sword and the Brush" process helps people to seamlessly transmute their struggles into positive results, using the sword to cut away old patterns and the brush to help paint the picture of the new life that they require.

Author of *More Truth Will Set You Free,* the Get a Grip series of pocket-size books, and several children's books, Derek has also hosted his own radio show, *The Way with Derek O'Neill,* which enjoyed the most successful launch in VoiceAmerica's history, quickly garnering 100,000 listeners.

Early in his career, Derek became involved with numerous charities in Ireland. Soon after traveling to India and witnessing the dire circumstances of countless people, he committed to devote his time, resources, and energy to alleviating unnecessary suffering around the world. He formed SQ Foundation, a not-for-profit organization, to provide food, medicine, water, education, and shelter to communities in need around the world. Currently operating in twelve countries and meeting the needs of hundreds of thousands of people, SQ Foundation seeks to identify projects and organizations with passionate leaders, often overlooked by larger institutions, where relatively small amounts of funds go a long way. In 2012, Derek was honored as Humanitarian of the Year and named International Celebrity Ambassador for Variety International the Children's Charity, and in 2013 he was named vice president of the charity.

Derek advises businesses, charities, celebrities, business leaders, and politicians, helping them to find new perspectives on long-standing issues and bringing harmony, growth, and high-performance back to their lives and businesses. Derek has worked with executives from some of the world's major airlines as well as the production team of *Spiderman on Broadway* to help the show become one of the most successful in the history of Broadway. He has been featured in *Exceptional People Magazine, The Irish Independent,* and *The Irish Examiner.* Recent television appearances include *CBS Good Day Sacramento* and a feature on *RTÉ,* Ireland's National TV Network.

To learn more about Derek O'Neill, to attend his next workshops, to order books, downloads, video broadcasts, or to contact him, please visit his website: www.derekoneill.com. To learn more about SQ Foundation, the global charity that is changing the lives of hundreds of thousands of people around the world, go to www.SQ-Foundation.org.

Jennifer Waldburger, MSW, earned her master's degree in social work from the University of Wisconsin-Madison, during which time she contributed to research with the Mayo Clinic. Jennifer, who has been working with children and families for more than fifteen years, is cofounder of Sleepy Planet, a company that offers education, parenting groups, and collaborative consultation to parents of babies and older children. Cocreator of the award-winning book and DVD *The Sleepeasy Solution,* Jennifer has been featured in a wide variety of media, including *Good Morning America, The Today Show, The CBS Evening News, Bringing Home Baby, The New York Times, The Wall Street Journal, The Los Angeles Times, Los Angeles Magazine, Variety, People, Parenting,* and *Parents.* Jennifer is also a consultant on NBC's hit show *The Pajanimals,* a joint production with the Jim Henson Company and Sprout, and is a featured expert and regular contributor for The Mother Company (themotherco.com). She is also cofounder of MomAssembly, an online "parenting university" for moms that offers video classes on a wide variety of parenting and lifestyle topics. For more information, visit www.sleepyplanet.com and www.momassembly.com.

Derek and Jennifer are contributors to the inspirational website PositivelyPositive.com and are co-creators of Calm Mama, Happy Baby, which provides supports and resources to moms and parents to help manage stress and create a calm, loving, and peaceful environment in which to raise their child. For more information, please visit www.calmandhappy.com.

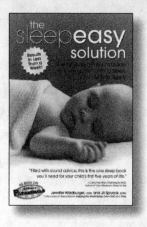